# Herbal Cattle Care For Homesteaders

*Using natural herbs for the prevention and treatment of cattle health concerns*

DR. AMANDA P. CARTWRIGHT

## Acknowledgments

I would like to thank Rick and Jane Austin for giving me a chance. You had faith in me and I will never be able to say thank you enough for the opportunity to be a speaker at Prepper Camp. Your kindness has opened many doors for me and I am very grateful. It is an honor to be your friend. (www.preppercamp.com)

Many thanks to Dr. Patrick Jones. Your knowledge and way of teaching is how I have learned herbs. I have learned more from you in your online herbal school than I ever did in all of my many years of graduate work to become a doctor of natural medicine. (https://bit.ly/3lo3YOd)

I am grateful to Jeremiah, my husband, who thinks I'm crazy (but I'm not the one who married me…) but still does this insane thing called life with me.

I am also appreciative to my sister, Rachel, for how you cope with your chaotic life as a mother, teacher, caretaker, and role model. You are definitely admired. I don't know how you don't break under all the pressure. You're a very strong individual.

And last but not least, to all the current and future world leaders, I hope you know what you are doing. I refuse to allow my freedom to be taken away because you cannot stand strong against money, control, and power. Stop lining your pockets to go along with corrupt agendas. Don't be manipulated. Learn from history. Grow some balls.

**Disclaimer**:

*The publisher and the author are providing this book and its contents on an "as is" basis and make no representations or warranties of any kind with respect to this book or its contents. The publisher and the author disclaim all such representations and warranties, including but not limited to warranties of healthcare for a particular purpose. In addition, the publisher and the author assume no responsibility for errors, inaccuracies, omissions, or any other inconsistencies (including citations) herein.*

*The content of this book is for informational purposes only and is not intended to diagnose, treat, cure, or prevent any condition or disease of an animal. You understand that this book is not intended as a substitute for consultation with a licensed veterinarian. Please consult with your own veterinarian regarding the suggestions and recommendations made in this book. The use of this book implies your acceptance of this disclaimer.*

*The publisher and the author make no guarantees concerning the level of success you may experience by following the advice and strategies contained in this book, and you accept the risk that results will differ for each animal.*

# CONTENTS

## About the Author

I am a Naturopathic physician. I am not a veterinarian. I have spent countless hours in my graduate studies training to treat and diagnose humans, but not animals. My eyes were opened to a different aspect of using herbal remedies with animals when I began taking courses through the Homegrown Herbalist School of Botanical Medicine. As a Naturopathic physician and veterinarian, Dr. Patrick Jones teaches online courses that are easy to understand and extremely helpful. You can take the lifetime access courses at your own pace and he is constantly adding more classes. I must say, I learned more from his school than I ever did in my doctorate of Naturopathic physician training. His herbology knowledge is impeccable and I highly recommend you going through his school. The knowledge you get will be something you can take and use for the rest of your life. That wisdom will not only help you and your family, but your animals as well. Plus, if you have questions, he will answer them on the school forums! I am an affiliate with his school, however even if I was not, I would still be highly recommending his school. Through the affiliate link listed below, you can also purchase premade tinctures and/or dried herbs if you prefer not to grow them yourself. They are very high quality. https://bit.ly/3lo3YOd

Another way my eyes were opened to using herbal medicine with animals is when my husband and I began a self-sufficient thriving homestead. When the 'plandemic' happened in 2020, my husband and I began understanding that we had to stop relying on other people because it could be taken away with a blink of an eye. We relied too much on the water company and the power company and the grocery store. So, we began learning and understanding how the land and animals can provide everything a person needs. All it takes is hard work and wisdom. I am thankful our eyes were opened to learn self-sufficiency and be able to implement it so we know what to do and expect in a SHTF scenario. In the process, we became homestead consultants which we have grown to love. Animals are a big part of living off the land and knowing how to handle their health issues is just another piece of the puzzle.

I am also an author of several books found in many bookstores in America. They are listed below.

Survival Herbs For Beginners: Herbal Medicine Made Easy

Boost Your Lazy Immune System: 6 Steps to Better Health and Wellness

Health Assessment and Exam: For Goats
https://a.co/d/0Cs6yiX

Health Assessment and Exam: For Rabbits
https://a.co/d/aujzRgz

The Following books are or will be published soon and are or will be available for purchase on Amazon, Books-A-Million, Barnes and Noble, and many other bookstores!

Herbal Horse Care for Homesteaders

Herbal Cat Care for Homesteaders

Herbal Dog Care for Homesteaders

Herbal Goat Care for Homesteaders

Herbal Rabbit Care for Homesteaders

Herbal Sheep Care for Homesteaders

Herbal Chicken Care for Homesteaders

Herbal Pig Care for Homesteaders

Herbal Duck Care for Homesteaders

Herbal Animal Care for Homesteaders:  A collection of all the books above!

I urge you to check out our YouTube channel called Survival Homestead Teaching Farm.  Subscribe and let us know if you have video suggestions!  We teach you about herbs, things that we have learned on our way to becoming homesteaders, and the knowledge to survive when SHTF happens. https://www.youtube.com/@survivalhomesteadteachingfarm

As if a doctor, author, consultant, and content creator wasn't enough, I am also an event speaker.  I absolutely love educating others at homesteading festivals and events.  I have been a speaker at Prepper Camp 2023 (www.preppercamp.com) in Saluda NC and look forward to speaking for as long as they let me.  I have also spoke at the Kentucky Sustainable Living Expo and look forward to speaking at other events including Mountain Readiness in Harmony NC (https://www.mountainreadiness.com/?ref=-NINwVjMEQq7ls) (Affiliate link), the East Tennessee Homestead Alliance in TN, and many other events too!

Enough about me….lets talk about herbs and cattle!  Some cattle information in this book may apply to you…some may not.  In the end, please take away knowledge that could be of help to you today, tomorrow, or in the future, whether you have the cattle currently or not.  You never know in a SHTF situation when you may need to barter your knowledge.

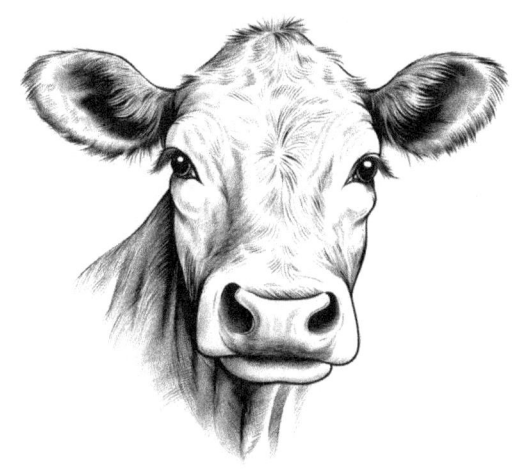

## Chapter 1:

## Homesteading

Having a homestead to allow complete freedom to live off the land and animals is not easy. A couple hundred years ago, people had to face incredible hardships to build a life. They had no choice because survival was ingrained in them from birth. They grew all their food, had to go to the nearby stream with buckets for all their water consumption and bathing, and figure out how to stay warm through terrible winters. There was a constant threat of disease, fear of being killed by wild animals, and incredible loneliness from being isolated on hundreds of miles of open land.

In modern day, people have become lazy. Most people don't have to work sun up to sun down outside in the scorching sun or in the dead of winter for their families to be fed. Instead, we purchase all our food from grocery stores, rely on the water company to always have water when you turn on the faucet, depend on electricity for heating and cooking, and rest upon knowing a veterinarian will always be a phone call away.

The worry in the past has been about how to stay fed, how to stay warm, and how to stay alive. Today, people have too much ease, too much comfort, and too much spare time. When we want something, we click a button on our phones and it arrives at our doorstep.

Fortunately, with the 'plandemic' (as I like to refer to it), many people are beginning to go back to the old ways where we rely on ourselves instead of others for everything needed for survival. Many are starting to see the grocery store prices surge, they are starting to see how unhealthy processed foods or even store-bought produce really is, and they are starting to follow the money trails and see just how big businesses are not in our best interest.

As homesteaders, we want a plot of land, a home of our own, good health, a community we are apart of, hope for our children, and a life filled with meaning and purpose. It's the same as what our ancestors wanted, but we must work hard to beat a system that has trained us to rely on others. We must slow down, reconnect with others, get out of our mind, and find inner piece with being one with our land and animals.

My husband and I chose to homestead for many reasons. The uncertainty of how the world is right now is one reason we homestead. We had a growing awareness of storm clouds on the horizon and could see things heading in the wrong direction. We made a choice to avoid catastrophe.

When anyone chooses a homesteading lifestyle, they are going against the mainstream culture. We realized we were in a culture addicted to digital screens, smart devices, and reliant upon others for food and water. We went to the grocery store for food, we drank the water from our tap, never realizing that could all be taken away at some point. That was the catalyst that jumpstarted our homesteading lifestyle. However, we have learned through all the trials and tribulations of the back breaking work, that we are better for it. Better individuals, because its healthy - both physically and mentally. Sunsets mean more, we are thankful for rain, we are grateful for livestock that provide us with so much, and we can truly lift our head and be closer with nature.

Despite what mainstream opinions lead a person to believe, a homestead offers a haven of hope. Believe it or not, your life can improve when you are out of reach of manmade objects and more in tune with nature. Less unhealthy pizza deliveries, less sleepless nights from the sound and lights of cars right outside your windows, and less asphalt and concrete everywhere you look; and more nature experiences such as the serenity of a deer drinking from a pond, a chicken cackling to announce a successful egg lay, or a fragile sprout of a green been pushing out of the soil in a newly planted garden bed.

On a homestead, you are a part of something bigger; a divine plan of problem solving and perseverance, one in which you are truly free. Free from a world, who many believe is on the verge of destruction.

Having farm animals is a part of homesteading. They can provide a vast array of different types of food including meat, eggs, and milk. On top of that, they provide tender memories that will stay with you for a lifetime. It's a humbling feeling, knowing they rely on you for everything, even love.

When faced with a medical crisis with your animals, you need to understand what to do to help. What medications does the animal need? What dosages? How do I get these medications? Sometimes there just is not time to call a veterinarian. What happens if you do not have the option to call a veterinarian?

Many livestock cannot be taken to your ordinary Veterinarian. Finding a Veterinarian that is knowledgeable in livestock, and willing to come to your homestead can be difficult to find and costly depending upon where you live.

Unfortunately, present day thoughts on medication go straight to pharmaceuticals. People seek out an instant fix with toxic chemicals and vaccines mostly due to lack of time to prepare their own medications for themselves and their animals, the lack of education of alternative remedies, and the power of persuasions of modern commercialism and advertisement. Many have been persuaded to believe artificial remedies is the best route, not realizing the information came from businesses who only have monetary profit in mind.

Cultivating your medications from your own land is not only an amazing, relatively inexpensive, tool for your animals but the fulfillment that you receive by having this knowledge can be accomplishing and satisfying. Being an animal owner means you must have an open mind and be eager to absorb new knowledge and ideas. Herbal comprehension is extensive and will take time to understand, but if you put the work in, it will pay off.

Herbs grow upon the earth for a reason. God put all the medicine on this earth that we as humans or your animals need without having to rely on pharmaceutical medications. Herbs are an important part of nature's chart of wholeness.

Sir Albert Howard, an agriculturist and scientist in the early 20th century, believed that man's neglect of medicinal plants is one of the basic causes of human and animal disease. Herbal medicine can result in remarkable cures.

In fact, pharmaceutical medications are a relatively new thing in the grand scheme of things. Homesteaders/farmers have been relying on herbal cures for thousands of years. We, as a society, have lost that knowledge because we started relying on other people to help instead of helping ourselves.

Animals have been using plants for healing purposes for centuries. It is from observing wild animals that humans learned the healing benefits of plants. For example, in the western United States, Indian tribes learned about the antimicrobial properties of Osha herb by observing bears ingest and roll in the plants.  Osha is mainly known and used by humans for its antiviral benefits. It is referred to by many as "bear medicine".

There are a number of other interesting discoveries including chimpanzees eating plants to settle their stomachs or chimps using medicinal plants more during the rainy season when they are more susceptible to pneumonia and other diseases. Monkeys even ingest plants to manage fertility including plants that contain isoflavonoids (a compound structurally similar to estrogen) after giving birth to reduce their fertility and when they are ready to give birth, they begin eating a plant called "monkeys ear" that produces a fertility enhancing steroid.

Have you ever noticed how dogs will know just what type of grass they need to eat when they have an upset stomach. They know how much they need and when to eat it.  Their dog parents didn't take them to the side and teach them this knowledge.  They just have an ability to know exactly what they need for the problem they are facing.

All animals, including your cattle, have an inherent ability to self-select specific plants for use against issues they are facing.  They not only know which plant to consume, but they also know how much of that plant to consume to achieve the desired result. This phenomenon is known as Zoopharmacognosy – the study of animals using plants to heal themselves.

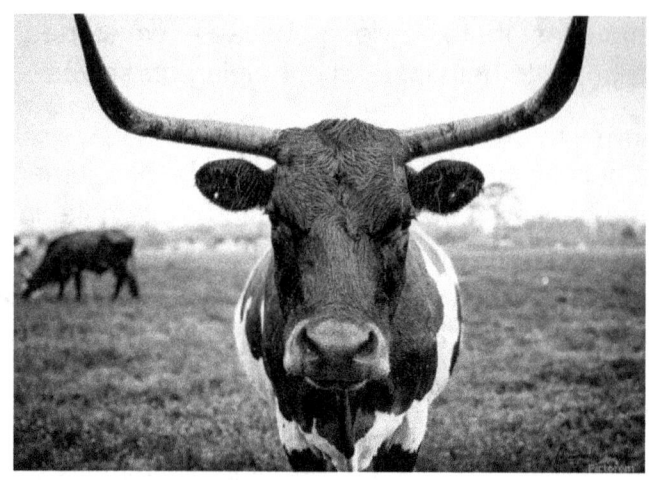

## Chapter 2:

## Why natural herbs over pharmaceuticals?

God put all the medicine on this earth that we as humans or your cattle need without having to rely on pharmaceutical medications. Herbs are an important part of nature and they focus on preventing and treating the root cause of health concerns in humans and cattle rather than merely alleviating the symptoms. This approach acknowledges that true healing and long-term well-being can only be achieved when we address the underlying causes of health concerns in your cattle.

Unlike the forceful action of pharmaceuticals medications, herbal medication nourishes your cattle's specific body system, aiding and assisting his/her body in healing itself. The benefits of herbal medicine are abundant and multifaceted. When you provide your cattle with an herbal remedy, your cattle often gets healthier due to their nourishing effects. This is not something that can generally be said for using pharmaceuticals with all their side effects (The Yale Ledger, 2022).

Synthetic medications are typically expensive and not always readily available. Herbs, on the other hand, are as inexpensive as a pack of seeds, and you can grow as many of them as you like and have room for in your yard.

You can grow your own medicine for your cattle. You can't grow pharmaceuticals, although many pharmaceuticals start out as an herbal form. It is then laced with chemicals so big companies can patent it and turn a profit.

Have you ever noticed how one medicine will hurt another function in the body and then you have to take another medicine to counteract the first medicines affects? It is a never-ending cycle. This is what the pharmaceutical companies want. They want you, or your cattle, to stay sick. Its more money in their pockets.

In order to understand the effectiveness of herbs, we must delve into the past and understand the history of herbs, veterinarians, and pharmaceuticals. Hundreds of years ago, the homesteader/farmer was an herbalist and a veterinarian all in one. They learned from a young age how to take care of their animals naturally because herbs were the only medicine.

This was knowledge that each person had long before there were doctors who solely took care of animals. None of those animals went extinct. They survived and thrived. So, what changed?

The use of plants as herbs has been important to all cultures since long before history was recorded. Hundreds of tribal cultures have used wild and cultivated herbs for medicinal and food purposes for thousands of years. As civilizations developed, so did the knowledge for the use of herbs (Coates, 2012).

Physicians in America studied and relied on plants as their primary medicines through the 1930s. Up until the 1930s, medical schools in America taught basic plant taxonomy, pharmacognosy, and medicinal plant therapeutics. Physicians routinely used plant drugs as their primary medicines. In fact, the word "drug" is derived from a word for the root of a plant.

In 1870 the United States Pharmacopoeia listed six hundred and thirty-eight herbs in its publication. By 1990 there were only fifty-eight herbs. Now, there are zero herbs listed (USP, 2023).

Some of these plants fell out of use due to their weakness or toxicity. However, the majority of clinically useful plants were replaced by pharmaceuticals which could be patented, thereby capable of generating larger profits as well as supporting conventional medicine (**PennState Extension, 2023**).

Herbal medicine is a vibrantly alive discipline that is being used actively in many other cultures throughout the world today. There is no question that herbal preparations can be of benefit to you or your cattle.

In France and Germany, it has been estimated that thirty to forty percent of all medical doctors/veterinarians rely on herbal preparations as their primary medicines. Unfortunately, the percentages in the United States are close to zero.

In the late 1700's veterinarian medicine began in France. In the mid 1800's, Americans became familiar with veterinarian medicine, however veterinarians were few and far between.

Up until 1965, all veterinarians in America used herbs as medicine to treat animals. It wasn't until 1965 that herbal medicine in the veterinarian practice was replaced by pharmaceuticals (Oakland Veterinary, 2019).

From 1965 to present day, pharmaceuticals have been sold to Americans, engraining it into them from birth, that toxic medications are the best and safest way of 'treating' health concerns. While I do agree some pharmaceuticals have their place, most should not be on the market, especially when there are natural herbs that can do the same thing. The food and drug administration states they are safe, however the lasting effects on the body are questionable.

Before the food and drug administration in 1965, veterinarians would fill their yards full of herbs so they would have medicine readily available when they needed. There were many benefits to treating animals in a very holistic and natural way. One of which was not having the side effects on the animal's liver as pharmaceuticals typically will enhance.

The liver filters all of the blood in the body and breaks down pharmaceuticals. If your cattle are on pharmaceutical medications, how do you know he or she will be able to metabolize those medications adequately? Why not give him/her herbs that you know their liver will be able to handle?

Along with your cattle's health, you must look of the bigger picture. Providing pharmaceutical medications to your cattle means there are pharmaceutical components in your soil. If you use their manure for compost, then you are putting those pharmaceutical components around your garden and then you are consuming those plants. Do you see the vicious cycle?

Another concern for pharmaceuticals is resistance. Antibiotics especially can become resistant with excessive usage. This means they will not work on your cattle when needed. They can, in turn, create gastrointestinal issues, palpitations, and/or seizures, all of which are unnecessary. Why put your cattle though pain when it could be avoided?

There are no doubts veterinarian bills are expensive. The national average veterinarian bill, consisting of only general routine maintenance for cattle, is over one thousand dollars a year. That is one big reason to go herbal.

Another reason is the fact that getting a veterinarian to come to your farm is a concern for many. You can't just load your cattle in your car and haul him to the vet like a dog or cat.

Veterinarians who can diagnose and treat large animals are few and far between.

Those may not be the only reasons you want to treat your cattle as naturally as possible. You may choose to go the herbal route for financial reasons. You may choose to go the herbal route for health benefits to your cattle. You may choose to go the herbal route because of how the world is changing and becoming so uncertain.

If you are tired of agendas being pushed, especially those in the pharmaceutical realm, consider going back to simpler times, before monetary profit was the biggest goal, and harness the knowledge of herbal medications for your cattle.

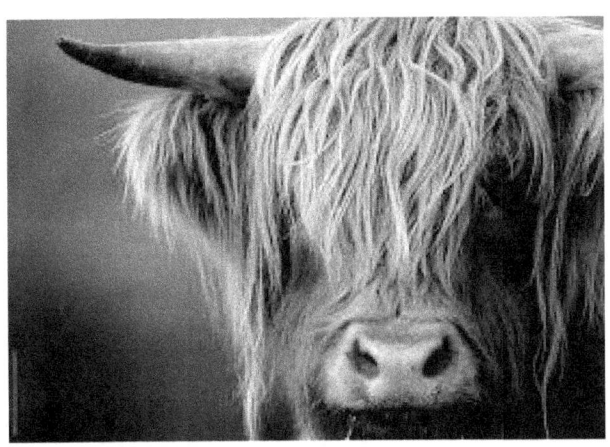

**Chapter 3:**

**Herbal Knowledge**

With herbal knowledge, you will be able to treat your cattle in times of crisis. If you are able, I would always recommend consulting a veterinarian but with how the world is currently changing, you never know when you will need this wisdom in your back pocket.

In June of 2023, the U.S. Food and Drug Administration mandated all medically important antimicrobials and other general livestock and pet medications to be removed from over-the-counter to prescription only by a qualified veterinarian.

Because of this change, many have been researching and understanding herbal medications better to use on their cattle for general use and for crisis situations. While many feel herbal medication is plan 'B', there are many others who have solely used herbal medications on their cattle for years and have had great success.

While herbal medications can be used as a preventative or to treat a particular ailment, if your cattle are taking any type of pharmaceuticals, you need to air on the side of caution because the herbs and pharmaceutical medication can and will interact with each other. Also, some herbs can be dangerous during pregnancy and lactation.

Herbs have many benefits over pharmaceuticals and are amazing medicine. Pharmaceuticals can be strong and have significant side effects. Using natural medications can reduce your animal's reliance on synthetic toxins and avoid possible side effects. Natural herbal medications are also more accessible. You can purchase dried herbs or grow them yourself. Once you have access to herbs, all you need is the knowledge of how and when to use them.

Wouldn't it be nice to be able to see a problem with your cattle, go to your yard and grab a twig of this of sprig of that, and treat your cattle without the costly veterinarian bills?

If you purchase dried herbs, you can expect a shelf life of around a year, more if you purchase from a reputable place such as from the Homegrown Herbal School of Botanical Medicine. https://bit.ly/3lo3YOd If you grow and dry an herb yourself, you can expect around a two-year shelf life but the way you dry the herb and store the herb does play a big role in that shelf life.

Ways to dry herbs include using a dehydrator, using a freeze drier, or simply using screens to air dry over several days. Whichever way you choose, make sure to keep the herbs away from direct sunlight and never dry it above one hundred-and ten-degrees Fahrenheit. This changes the chemical bonds and 'cooks' the herb, making the medicinal benefits disappear. Always wait to grind the herb into a powder until you are ready to use it. This helps keep the medicinal properties intact and prolongs the shelf life.

Depending on your cattle, some herbs may be best used fresh. Some herbs are meant to be used short term and some herbs are meant to be used for a longer term. If your cattle have chronic problems and they are consuming an herb long term, it is best to give their body a rest. Every couple of weeks, take a day off and do not give the herb to your cattle. This will allow their body to reset. Usually when they resume consuming the herb, the herb works even better at combating the particular ailment.

How much of an herb to give depends on your cattle and their needs. It also depends on many other factors such as gender, weight, age, the actual herb, and other foods/medications he or she is already consuming. The dosing listed in this book, except for calves, is based upon an average one-thousand-pound healthy adult cow/bull.

Some cattle are harder than others to get to consume herbal medicine. For livestock, fresh herbs are usually eaten without a second thought and dried powdered herbs mixed into their feed works most of the time. But what about finnicky cattle? Sometimes you have to be creative when it comes to giving your cattle herbal medicine by mixing it in with their normal feed, making a tea and adding that to their water bucket, making a tincture and adding a few drops to their feed or water, making an herbal oil or salve and rubbing that into a wound or stiff joint, or simply hiding the herb in something delicious they enjoy eating. We will discuss more about teas, tinctures, herbal oils, poultices, and salves in chapter five.

I must not fail to mention that consuming herbs is not the only route of administration. Topical use can also be applied when the situation allows.

Many of the herbs mentioned in chapter 8 can be grown in your yard alongside your decorative flowers. Many of them are perennial so once you plant them, you don't have to worry about saving the seeds and replanting them year after year. Your yard can be full of medicine, but look like a regular flower garden to most.

Planting herbs for your cattle can also create a bonus that will allure pollinating bees towards your property and potentially your gardens. The herbs look nice but have functionality too!

## Safety

There have been some controversial rumors about the effectiveness and safety of herbs. Obviously, if your cow is pregnant or one of your cattle are taking other pharmaceutical medication, be cautious with giving herbs internally.

Comfrey is one herb that has gotten a bad rap in the past few decades. It works really well, however there are many research studies that show how ineffective it may be to your cattle. You must take a look at the type of study and how the study was administered to understand herbs, specifically comfrey (Mount Sinai, n.d.).

In one study, six-week-old rats were fed comfrey as forty percent of their diet and some of those rats developed liver tumors. If you ate only one particular food as forty percent of your diet, without getting other needed vitamins, minerals, and nutrients, you would have problems too!

What the studies failed to do is let us know other factors that could have contributed to the liver tumors. What pharmaceuticals were the rats on at the time of the study? What did the rats diet consist of? Were they ingesting other food additives? How healthy were the rats' livers prior to the study? We don't know because the study didn't take all the factors into consideration. Scientists can say 'research says….' and most of the time people fall for it.

I think it is safe to say that cattle should not consume comfrey as forty percent of our diet. I also think it would be wise to not give comfrey to your cattle internally at excessively high doses (more than forty leaves per day) or for prolonged periods of time. I would not think negatively about comfrey based on research studies that are not taking all factors into account. Look at the many positive comfrey testimonials of cattle owners and draw your own conclusion.

Comfrey isn't the only controversial herb. Many websites claim herbs are unsafe because research on that particular herb is lacking. To be very honest, there are hundreds of years of research with these herbs. Just look at history! Herbs were the medicine of our ancestors and the medicine they gave their livestock to keep them healthy. Maybe looking back on history will help some understand the safety and effectiveness of herbs for their cattle.

Many scientific sources claim herbs are bad, only to find out in the end that some scientists are paid to say this in order to push pharmaceutical medications which puts money into certain people's pockets.

It is true that some herbs can cause allergic reactions. The pharmaceuticals do too! With giving herbs to your cattle, you need to have a bit of education to know how the herb will affect your cattle, proper dosage, and how to prevent the health concern in the first place. This is what this book aims to do!

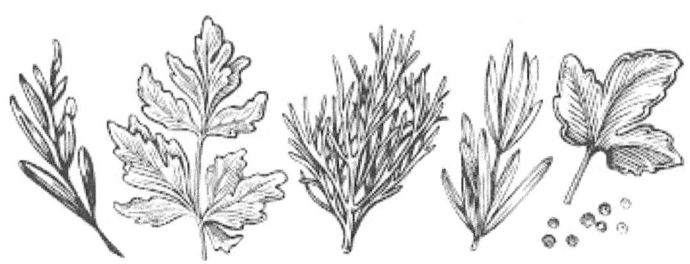

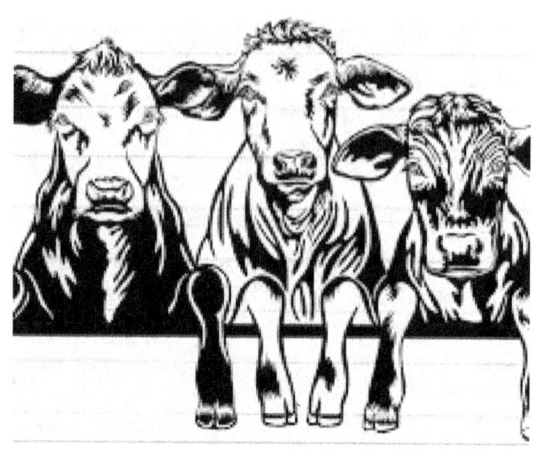

**Chapter 4:**

**How to harvest & dry herbs**

Of course, you can purchase herbs. If you do, make sure it is from a reputable place where you know how the herbs have been dried, how long they have been sitting on the shelf, and under what conditions have they been on the shelf. I mentioned the link for the Homegrown Herbalist at the beginning of this book. I do highly recommend them.

If you choose to grow your own herbs, you can have a natural pharmacy just outside your door, many of which will come back year after year. How fantastic would it be to open your door and have your own veterinarian pharmacy at your fingertips? Whether you grow medicinal herbs for cattle or you grow herbs as a deterrent for many pests, preventing and treating naturally can potentially save you hundreds of dollars on veterinarian bills and possibly save your cattle a lot of hassle with having toxic pharmaceuticals running through their system.

It is best to harvest herbs early in the day, after the dew is gone, but before the hot sun can dry out the oils inside the herb. Only harvest some of the plant to make sure it doesn't die.

If you are harvesting leaves, you will usually cut off small branches, making it easier to dry them. For flowers, wait until they have developed fully and harvest them as soon as possible after they have fully opened. If you are harvesting only the seeds, you will need to wait until the seeds mature and the seed pod dries on the stem before harvesting.

Once you have the herb, you may want to dry the herbs for later use. There are a few ways this can be accomplished. Traditionally, herbs are air-dried without any additional heat source. Many choose to bundle the herb together by tying the stems with string or a rubber band and hanging them upside-down in a dry place away from light.

Drying racks are another option. This is another way to allow air to dry the herbs for three to four weeks without adding heat or allowing light to penetrate the herb.

It is possible to dry herbs with a dehydrator. Ideally it should have a fan to circulate the warm air so that the entire batch dries evenly. You must make sure the temperature setting is not at or above one-hundred- and ten-degrees Fahrenheit. Drying at or above this temperature will kill all the medicinal benefits. This is another reason you must do your due diligence on finding a reputable herb company if purchasing without growing yourself. You need to know how the herb has been dried and how long it has been sitting on the shelf!

Store your dried herbs in a clean, sealed glass jar away from light. Make sure they are one hundred percent dried before storing. As mentioned before, it is best to wait and crush them into a powder until immediately before using the herb for your cattle.

In order to powder the herbs, simply take the herbs and crush with a blender or mash them using a hand-held mortar and pestle.  Some may choose to use a spice-mill or coffee bean grinder.  Afterwards, you may want to use a fine sieve to make sure everything has been pulverized into a fine powder.  This is not one hundred percent needed for your cattle, but it may help when making herbs into teas, tinctures, herbal oils, herbal salves, etc.

Even if you don't have the space or simply don't want to grow these herbs, look at the amount of money you would save by purchasing already dried and powdered herbs that ship right to your door versus a veterinarian bill.  Of course, if you decide to purchase herbs, you need to make sure they are from a reputable source.

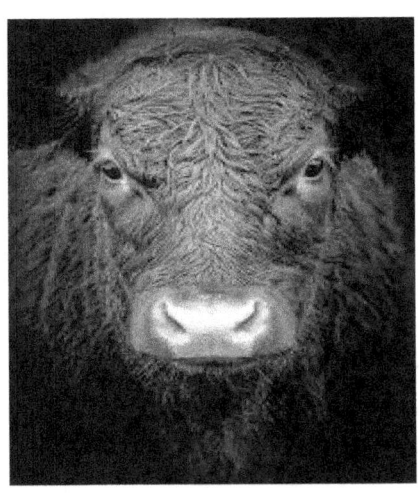

**Chapter 5:**

**How to use herbs medicinally**

When it comes to herbal medicine, there is no shortage of options for reaping the bountiful benefits of these natural wonders. From tinctures to salves, a poultice, oils, and teas, each delivery method offers a unique way to harness the healing powers of medicinal herbs that promote overall well-being.

Once you have those herbs dried and powdered, what do you do with them? Sometimes your cattle will enjoy the new taste and devour it without giving you grief. Sometimes you might not get so lucky. There are many ways to process herbs. I'll take you through a few steps briefly so you will know exactly what to do.

## Herbal infusions/decoctions (Tea)

A tea, also known as an infusion or decoction is taking an herb and infusing it into water. Using an herbs' leaves or flower is called and infusion and using the bark or stems in a more concentrated form of an herb is called a decoction. There are several methods to use and you can infuse more than one herb at a time if desired (Apelian, 2021).

To give an herbal tea to a cow/bull, simply allow it to drink the tea. If they seem to not want to drink it, you can always add it to their water bucket in increments. If neither of these options work, you can syringe it into the back of their throat.

Stove method:

1.      To make an infusion, start with cold distilled or purified water in a non-metal cooking pot with a lid. The cold water ensures the maximum amount of beneficial nutrients from the herb(s) are extracted. Use a ratio of four-ounces dried herb(s) to sixty-four ounces water. Let it soak for a few hours in the cold water.

2.      Cover the cooking pot and boil slowly. It must be covered to allow all medicinal benefits to stay inside. Once it begins to boil, decrease the temperature to simmer fifteen to twenty minutes or until the volume of the liquid has reduced to thirty-two ounces.

3.      Strain with a cheesecloth and let it cool. Squeeze herb(s) through the cheesecloth to ensure all liquid has been removed. Pour into a clean glass jar with a lid. This can be stored in the refrigerator for up to two days or it can be frozen.

Cup Method:

1.      Place one ounce of your herb(s) into a sixteen-ounce mug.

2.      Pour boiling water over the top.

3.      Place a lid, plate, or anything you have over the top of the mug.  This is very important.  This keeps all the medicinal benefits inside the cup and prevents them from escaping.

4.      Allow this to simmer for at least ten minutes but preferably up to two hours.

5.      Remove the lid and strain the herb(s).

6.      Use with your cattle immediately.


French Press Method:

1.      Place two ounces of your herb(s) into a French press.

2.      Insert the strainer part on your French press with strainer part to the top.

3.      Pour thirty-two ounces boiling water over the top of your herb(s).

4.      Place the lid on the top of the French press but do not push down on the strainer.  Leave it up.

5.      Allow this to simmer for at least ten minutes but preferably up to two hours.

6.      After this period of time, push down on the strainer to allow all the herb(s) to be pushed to the bottom of the French press.

7.      Allow the tea to cool before giving to your cattle.


Tincture

A tincture is a concentrated liquid herbal extract obtained by steeping dried herbs in alcohol.  The alcohol breaks down the plant's cell walls, liberating its bioactive compounds, which are then preserved in the alcohol solution (Apelian, 2021).

To preserve the dried herb(s) indefinitely, the alcohol used should be eighty to one hundred-proof.  Vodka is usually the cheapest, has no flavor, and is usually preferred in a tincture, however other alcohols can be used as long as it is at least eighty-proof.

Over the course of four to eight weeks, the dried herb(s) infuses into the alcohol. Some will say differently; however, with a tincture, you always want to use dried herbs, whether they are powdered or not. The moisture content of fresh herbs can damage the longevity of the preservation (Apelian, 2021).

It is worth noting the differences between a tincture and an extract. A tincture uses alcohol whereas an extract uses other liquids such as apple cider vinegar or glycerin. An extract does not have the shelf life of a tincture.

When making tinctures, you can put several herbs into the jar with the eighty to one hundred proof alcohol. However, if you have several different tinctures already made up, you can't add that to the tincture you are making.

To give a tincture internally to cattle, merely place a few drops into their water bucket or use as directed by the particular ailment they are facing. Most people know that tinctures are taken internally but did you know they can be used externally as well?

Topical use of tinctures can help your cattle with various wounds, bites, and stings. The amber bottles made for tinctures do sometimes come with spray tops. You put the spray top on the bottle and spray the tincture directly onto the wound, bite, or sting.

One caveat to spraying a tincture is watering it down. Watering the tincture down will help the wound to not burn as much when applying the tincture. If you do water it down, make sure to use good, clean water. I prefer soft rain water. Do not ever use tap water. This is laced with many harmful chemicals. Once you add water to the tincture, it should be used up completely within two days. Add water at a ratio of one part tincture to five parts water.

To give a tincture to cattle, you can add it to their feed or you can add a small amount of clean water and syringe it into the back of their throat.

There are two methods of making tinctures.

Folk Method:

1.     Fill a clean glass jar half full of the dried herb(s) you are using.

2.     Fill jar with alcohol leaving a half inch headspace in the jar.

3.     Alcohol (or anything acidic) tends to rust metal lids, therefore if you place a piece of wax paper or parchment paper under the lid before screwing it on, it will keep a barrier there to help avoid rusting.

4.     Once the lid is on, turn it up-side-down to mix well.

5.     Label the jar with the herb(s) used and date the tincture is started.

6.     Keep the jar in a cool, dry, dark location for eight weeks to six months, shaking it daily to mix.

7.     After this time period, strain out the herb through a cheesecloth.

8.     Pour tincture into an amber color bottle.  The amber color bottles keep light from entering the bottle.  Light will denature a tincture and cause the shelf life to shorten.

Ratio Method: (1 to 5)

1.     Using a scale, set a clean glass jar on top and press 'tare'.  This will allow you to measure the exact quantity of herb(s) and alcohol to use.

2.    Use one part herb(s) to five parts alcohol in the glass jar. (This method helps save alcohol and makes the tinctures more consistent from batch to batch) Example: If you use five grams herb(s), use twenty-five grams alcohol.

3.    Alcohol (or anything acidic) tends to rust metal lids, therefore if you place a piece of wax paper or parchment paper under the lid before screwing it on, it will keep a barrier there to help avoid rusting.

4.    Once the lid is on, turn it up-side-down to mix well.

5.    Label the jar with the herb(s) used and date the tincture is started.

6.    Keep the jar in a cool, dry, dark location for eight weeks to six months, shaking it daily to mix.

7.    After this time period, strain out the herb through a cheesecloth.

8.    Pour tincture into an amber color bottle. The amber color bottles keep light from entering the bottle. Light will denature a tincture and cause the shelf life to shorten.

Herbal Oil Infusion

Herbal oil infusions are carrier oils that have had dried herbs soaked in them for a period of time. These are then used topically on your cattle. The herbs must be dried because the moisture content of fresh herbs could make the oil go rancid. Herbal infused oils can keep for one to two years if stored properly (Apelian, 2021).

Carrier oils are plant-based oils used to 'carry' the medicinal benefits of an herb onto the cattle's skin. These carrier oils that are good for cattle skin are organic olive oil, sweet almond oil, coconut oil, emu oil, jojoba oil, castor oil, tamanu oil, grapeseed oil, argon oil, apricot oil, avocado oil, lard (from pigs), and tallow (from cattle).

Please do not confuse an herbal infused oil with an essential oil. Essential oils are the oils naturally found in an herb which are extracted. It takes very large amounts of an herb to make a very small amount of essential oil. Essential oils are highly concentrated and so powerful that they should almost never be applied directly to cattle's skin.

Cold Herbal Oil Infusion Method:

1.    In a clean glass jar, fill half way with dried herb(s).

2.    Pour a carrier oil over the herb. Fill within a half inch of the top.

3.    Put lid onto the jar.

4.    Mix well by turning the jar up-side-down.

5.    Label the jar with the herb(s) used, carrier oil used, and the date.

6.    For six to eight weeks, keep the jar in a location away from light and turn it up-side-down at least once a day to mix the herb(s) and carrier oil.

7.    After the six to eight weeks, remove the lid and strain the herb(s) through a cheesecloth. Squeeze the cheesecloth to get all the oil out.

8.    Store in a clean glass jar with a lid in a cool, dry, dark location and label with the herb(s), carrier oil used, and date of completion. You can use immediately on your cattle by applying topically to wounds. You can also use this to make an herbal salve.

Hot Herbal Oil Infusion Method: Crockpot

1.    In a clean glass jar, fill half way with dried herb(s).

2.    Pour a carrier oil over the herb. Fill within a half inch of the top.

3.    Put lid onto the jar.

4.    Mix well by turning the jar up-side-down.

5.    Put the jar or jars into a crockpot with a 'warm' setting.

6.    Add about two inches of water to the crockpot. Add more water when necessary to make sure the water level stays consistent throughout the entire process.

7.    Allow the jars to sit in the slightly warm crockpot water for four to seven days.

8.    Remove the jars from the crockpot and allow them to cool.

9.    Strain the herb(s) by using a cheesecloth. Squeeze all the carrier oil out.

10.    Put a lid on and label the jar with the herb(s) used, carrier oil used, and the date of completion. You can use immediately on your cattle by applying topically to wounds. You can also use this to make an herbal salve.


Hot Herbal Oil Infusion Method: Double Boiler

1.    Fill a cooking pot half way with water and bring to a boil.

2.    Add your herb(s) and carrier oil to a double boiler and set this on the top of the boiling water. Use a ratio of one part herb(s) to two parts carrier oil.

3.    Turn down the heat of the water and allow the mixture to simmer for four to five hours.

4.    Once the herb(s) have been thoroughly infused into the oil, strain the herb(s) out of the carrier oil through a cheesecloth. Squeeze the cheesecloth to get all the oil out.

5.    Put a lid on and label the jar with the herb(s) used, carrier oil used, and the date of completion. You can use immediately on your cattle by applying topically to wounds.

You can also use this to make an herbal salve. While this is a faster method, the crockpot method is still highly recommended.

Herbal Salve:

An herbal salve acts the same as an herbal oil infusion, except it takes on a solid substance that is easier to apply topically to cattle's wounds, skin irritations, or sore muscles. Vitamin E is commonly used in salves to help with rancidity problems; however, it is not a necessary ingredient. You must have an herbal infused oil to make a salve.

Containers that you use for your herbal salve should not be plastic or aluminum. Plastic can melt when you add the salve and it also can seep harmful chemicals into the salve. Aluminum does the same. Aluminum can cause brain, liver, and kidney problems in cattle so it is best to avoid it when possible.

1.      Fill a cooking pot half way with water and bring to a warm simmer (not boiling because you don't want to heat the herbal oil any more than one hundred degrees).

2.      Place one cup of your herbal infused oil into a double boiler on the top of the water.

3.      Add one fourth cup of beeswax.

4.      Add vitamin E oil at this time if desired.

5.      Once the beeswax has melted, mix well and add to your containers.

6.      Allow to cool completely to solidify.

Poultice

A poultice can be an effective way of getting a fresh or dried herb to soak into the skin quickly. A poultice is a common topical treatment used on cattle, usually used on the lower legs, to help inflammation, wounds, and to pull our toxins from bees, wasps, spiders, or snakes (Apelian, 2021).

A poultice needs to be wrapped to stay in place. A popular type of bandage to keep poultices in place is called Coflex. Coflex is a bandage material that wraps around an area that sticks to itself. Poultices needs to be changed frequently.

Traditional Method:

1.  Cut or crush the herb(s) up finely. You can do this with a knife, blender, or a mortar and pestle.

2.  Mix with a touch of water to create a mush mixture.

3.  Apply a generous quantity directly onto the cattle's skin.

4.  Wrap with a dressing. Change this dressing frequently.


Spit Method:

1.  Put several leaves of the herb(s) you are using in your mouth.

2.  Chew the herbs to a mush and spit out.

3.  Apply a generous quantity directly onto the cattle's skin.

4.  Wrap with a dressing. Change this dressing frequently.


Using herbs medicinally is as easy as feeding your cattle fresh or dried herbs, making an herbal infusion or decoction tea, preparing an herbal infused oil, making an herbal salve, producing a ready to go tincture, or making an on-demand poultice. In this book, fresh or powdered herbs are mainly mentioned for internal use, but you can use these in other forms such as tinctures or herbal infusions. Knowing how to use herbs medicinally is a big part of understanding herbal cattle care.

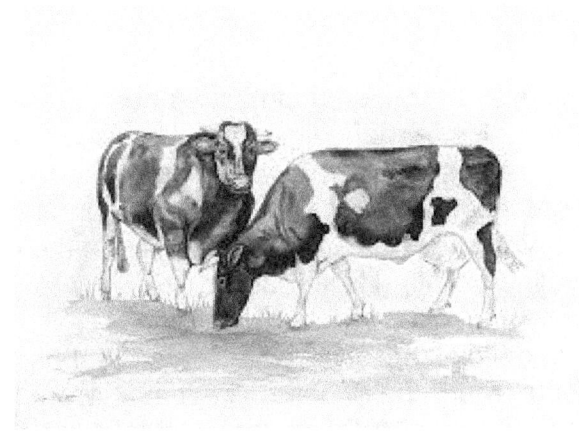

## Chapter 6:

## Immune System

The immune system is something that needs to be boosted with any type of cattle illness.  It is so important that it needs its own chapter.

The immune system of cattle are fascinating, complex, and plays a critical role in tackling the infections that it encounters. It is instrumental in protecting the cattle when foreign invaders, such as viruses, parasites, fungi, or bacteria, breach the physical barriers—such as skin and mucous membranes—and enter the body.

Chronic stress, whether physical or mental, weakens the immune system.  Age and nutrition are both also closely linked to immunity and immune function.  The following vitamins, minerals, and herbs can help boost your cattle's immune system.

## Vitamin A

Vitamin A plays a key role in maintaining healthy maintenance of cattle's eyes, skin, and the linings of the respiratory, digestive, and reproductive tracts.  It's also essential for proper functioning of the kidneys, and normal development of bones, teeth, and nerve tissue.  Vitamin A comes from the carotene in green and yellow plants (Nickel, 2020).

Early signs of deficiencies in vitamin A are night blindness, loss of appetite, rough hair coat, dull eyes, slowed gains, and reduced feed efficiency. Animals that are deficient can have lower fertility and reduced calving percentages (Nickel, 2020).

Because vitamin A is stored in the liver, symptoms of a deficient daily intake may not express themselves for as long as one hundred days (Nickel, 2020).

Depending on the environment, cattle consuming a diet of diverse, green forages year-round could potentially receive all the vitamin A they need.  To supplement, feed your cattle free choice of cantaloupe, bell peppers, and carrots which are all high in vitamin A (Nickel, 2020).

## Vitamin B1 (Thiamine)

Thiamine deficiency in beef cattle results in a fluid filled (edema) brain disorder that causes partial paralysis in the animal's ability to rise.  In attempts to rise, the ankles of the rear legs remain flexed.   Prolonged pressure caused by the edema causes damage to the brain usually without recovery. A drastic change in the animal's diet from low roughage (short grass) to grain supplements without hay commonly causes a deficiency (Beef Cattle, 2019).

## Vitamin B 12

Vitamin B12 is essential in cattle for energy metabolism and the production of red blood cells. Signs of deficiency include anemia, scaly ears, and a reduced appetite. They can also have a rough coat, reduced milk production, and be seen eating bark, leaves, or dirt. Things that effect vitamin b12 are soil, pasture, rainfall, age, and parasites (Agriculture and Food, 2019).

Unfortunately, there are no plants that produce specific vitamin b12. Therefore, microorganisms in the gut are the only natural source of vitamin b12. It is imperative the cattle graze on good grass and have a healthy diet to maintain the good active bacterial microorganisms in the gut (Pubmed, 2020).

## Vitamin D

Vitamin D is necessary for proper bone formation, maintaining calcium and phosphate in the body, preventing milk fever, and is required for the activation of critical innate immune defenses of cattle against microbial pathogens (Nelson, 2014).

A key issue to be aware of is that when vitamin D intake is less than adequate, the vitamin D-dependent functions of the immune system may be impaired even though the animal does not have symptoms of classical vitamin D deficiency (rickets, slow growth, stiffness) (Nelson, 2014).

In that condition of vitamin D insufficiency, cattle may be vulnerable to infectious diseases and may not be reaching peak production. Therefore, it is critical to make sure your cattle are getting enough vitamin D3 from direct sunlight (Bailey, 2017).

Vitamin D3 is made by the cattle's body when they are exposed to sunlight, however cattle also need vitamin D2. Vitamin D2 comes from plant sources that have been exposed to the sunlight. Many of these types of plants/herbs should be readily available for cattle consumption. They include small amounts of alfalfa grass daily, one cup of oyster and/or button mushrooms daily (although many cattle do not prefer their taste), two cups parsley daily, two cups thyme daily, and free choice of nettle leaves and dandelion greens (Mendicino, 2023).

## Vitamin E

Vitamin E is an important antioxidant that interacts with selenium to provide protection to cells and tissues and is involved with immune function. Vitamin E is soluble in fat stored by the body in adipose tissue and the liver. This is important, as it means that vitamin E does not need to be supplied daily to cattle (McKinnon, 2014).

Herbs high in vitamin E that can be fed daily include one half tablespoon of ground cayenne pepper per seven hundred pounds, one half cup oregano, five cups dried basil, and two cups dried parsley (Cooke, 2015).

## Calcium

Calcium is a naturally occurring element in water, soil, and rocks. Plants absorb calcium to support the structure of their cell walls and membranes. It is an integral part of bone and nerve tissue in cattle. Most well-managed pastures with legumes and alfalfa will have adequate calcium (PennState Extension, n.d.).

The most important feature of calcium nutrition is the ratio of calcium to phosphorus. The ideal calcium to phosphorus ratio is two parts calcium to one part phosphorus. If the ration is inverted and phosphorus exceeds calcium, absorption of calcium in the digestive tract is reduced and the animal will metabolize calcium and phosphorus from bone. This can result in less bone growth, brittle bones, or kidney stones (PennState Extension, n.d.).

Signs of calcium deficiency include anorexia, confusion, subnormal body temperature, cold extremities, low heart rate, decreased intensity of heart sounds, weak peripheral pulse, and inability to urinate (Partners in reproduction, n.d.).

A good source of calcium is limestone (PennState Extension, n.d.). Herbal sources of calcium include free choice of nettle, dandelion greens, oat straw, and plantain, along with two cups chamomile and five cups basil daily (Mendicino, 2023).

## Phosphorus

Phosphorus is a naturally occurring mineral in the earth. Plants absorb phosphorus from the earth and in return give cattle's bodies strong bones, good health and wellbeing, and it contributes to cattle's development.

Signs of cattle deficient in phosphorus include poor appetite, poor growth, high breeder mortality rates, reduced fertility and milk production, bone breakage, bone deformities, and peg leg. (MLA, n.d.).

Plants that are rich in phosphorus for cattle include daily free choice of stinging nettle, purslane, shepherd's purse, borage, and sunflowers (National Kidney Foundation, n.d.).

## Potassium

Most forages are adequate in potassium content and the needs of grazing cattle are generally met.  Potassium regulates fluid balance and blood pressure, maintains heart and kidney function, helps contract muscles, and transmits nerve signals.  (PennState Extension, n.d.).

Signs of potassium deficiency include depression, muscular weakness, stiffness, decreased feed intake, reduced heart rate, and nervousness (Better Crops, 1998).

Herbs high in potassium include daily free choice alfalfa and dandelion and four cups each of nettle and horsetail daily (St. Lukes Hospital, n.d.).

## Magnesium

Magnesium is an important mineral for grazing cattle because of the association with grass tetany. Grass tetany is usually seen in cattle in the early spring when there is lush grass growth and cool, wet weather and is caused by a deficiency of magnesium to the cattle.  The disease is characterized by a staggering gait, nervousness, and death of the animal.  It usually occurs in older cows, and death can result in a matter of hours after the onset of symptoms (PennState Extension, n.d.).

In the most acute form of hypomagnesemia tetany, affected cows, which may appear to be grazing normally, suddenly throw up their heads, bellow, gallop in a blind frenzy, fall, and exhibit severe paddling seizures with chomping of the jaws, frothy salivation, fluttering of the eyelids, and nystagmus. Seizures may recur at short intervals, and death usually occurs within a few hours (Stewart, 2022).

In less severe cases, twitching of the muscles of the face, flank, and shoulder may occur. The cow is obviously ill at ease, walks stiffly, is hypersensitive to touch and sound, urinates frequently, and may progress to the acute convulsive stage after a period as long as two to three days (Stewart, 2022).

When a cow is lactating, one tablespoon of coriander herbal oil will help increase magnesium levels. Also beneficial is a handful of dill, one cup of celery seed, and five cups of dried basil leaves (Stewart, 2022).

## Zinc

Zinc is a crucial trace element that plays a vital role in various physiological functions, including immune function, growth, and reproduction in livestock. Zinc deficiency can lead to various health problems in cattle, such as decreased growth rates, impaired reproductive performance, and increased susceptibility to diseases. In contrast, supplementing livestock diets with zinc can promote health and enhance microbiome balance, leading to improved animal welfare and productivity (Duffy, 2023).

High in zinc, the following herbs are good daily for cattle to increase zinc levels. Two cups parsley, five cups dried basil leaves, half of a cup of oregano leaves, two cups dried thyme, and two cups rosemary leaves (Duffy, 2023).

## Selenium

Selenium is an important trace element that is found in the soil and taken up by plants. Cattle consume selenium with the plants they eat. It is stored for a short period in the body, mainly in the liver. It acts in conjunction with vitamin E to protect cell membranes including cell walls. This protection is particularly important in muscle cells that work hard and consume large quantities of energy and oxygen (Agriculture and Food, 2019).

When there is a deficiency of selenium, harmful free radicals are generated. These damage skeletal muscle tissues of the heart and limbs. It is also very important in maintaining a healthy immune system so deficient cattle may be more susceptible to some common infectious diseases (Agriculture and Food, 2019).

Signs of deficiency include lowered milk production, lowered fertility, mastitis, premature and weak calves, perinatal death, abortions, muscular dystrophy, stiff legged gait, weakness, unable to stand or walk, and/or sudden death within two to three days. Even with deficiencies, it is rare simply because the amount cattle need is very low. Plants containing more than five parts per million is considered toxic to cattle (Agriculture and Food, 2019).

Plants that have selenium in them, but not at toxic levels, include wheatgrass, barley, wheat, and alfalfa. If the cattle have access to at least one of these grasses, usually the selenium levels are optimal (USDA, n.d.).

**Echinacea** (purpurea)

Echinacea, also known as coneflower, are native to North America. Echinacea is used to stimulate the immune system to resist infection in cattle. Two large handfuls daily of echinacea would suffice to boost their immune system (Progressive Dairy, 2020).

## Garlic

Garlic is an immune stimulant that acts to suppress bacterial, fungal and viral illness in cattle. (Progressive Dairy, 2020). It also reduces methane production, improves uptake of nutrients, improves general health and growth, and is an antibacterial. Twelve cloves of garlic daily would boost their immunity and help with any possible parasites (Groot, n.d.).

## Walnut

The leaves and hulls of black walnuts from the black walnut tree, activates the immune system and prevents diseases. (Groot, n.d.).

## Turmeric

Turmeric has been used for over four thousand years in India and has been proven very safe in cattle. It can help boost the immune system and maintain overall health (Groot, n.d).

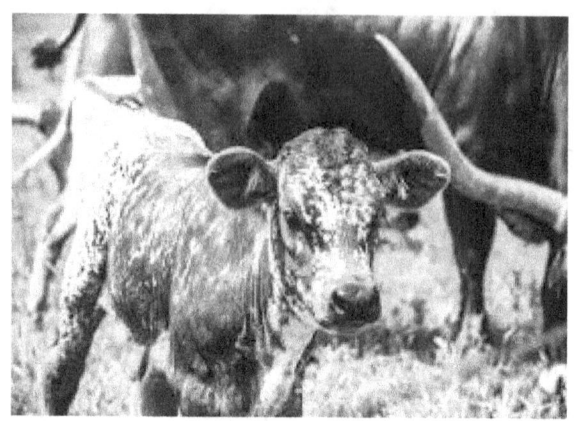

## Chapter 7:

## General cattle information and management

Cattle bring a variety of benefits to homesteads, whether by raising for milk, meat, hides, using to pull plows and carts, or using their manure as fertilizer.

Cattle belong to the family bovidae (bovine) and are one of the most commonly domesticated large farm animals. They can weigh up to four thousand pounds and be between five and a half feet and eight feet in length on average. Cattle are herbivores, so their diet consists mainly of pasture grass and hay (Understanding Animal Research, n.d.).

The male and female baby cattle are called calves. Baby females are called heifers and baby males are called bulls. Adult females are called cows and the adult males are called bulls if left fully intact. If the adult male is castrated, he is called a steer (Britannica, 2023).

Cattle are raised primarily for either beef or dairy. Beef cattle will yield on average five hundred pounds of de-boned meat for freezing. Dairy cows can produce six to seven gallons of milk daily when milked two to three times a day (Animal Welfare Institute, n.d.).

Like any animal, cattle require daily preventative care. I can't stress the importance of this enough. Preventative care is not only herbal care but it also consists of good feed, dry and well-ventilated housing, clean bedding, proper fencing, lots of pasture to exercise, etc. (Spaulding, 2010).

A daily check of your cattle is a key part of good care. If you notice any problems, such as lack of appetite, weight loss, diarrhea, constipation, swellings, or other unusual symptoms, give the animal a thorough examination at once. Tomorrow may be too late. Of course, this is easier said than done if you have lots of acreage and many cattle to care for on your homestead (Spaulding, 2010).

With any type of animal, you will have to face a health concern at some point. The best way to prevent that health concern from happening is by staying on top of what your cattle really need; however, sometimes ailments happen whether there were prevention protocols in place or not. Regular attention, good general care, and routine checkups are the keys to healthy cattle and happy animal owners (Spaulding, 2010).

**Housing**

Cattle are more likely to become sick due to too much shelter rather than too little. A barn with an opening to the south where the cattle wander in and out at will is a great option (Spaulding, 2010).

For specifically dairy cows, they should have individual bedded stalls inside the barn to help keep them cleaner (Spaulding, 2010).

It is very important to keep calves separate from each other until they are past weaning age. This prevents them from passing bacteria back and forth to each other, lessening the chance of an outbreak of calf scours or pneumonia (Spaulding, 2010).

## Feeding/Water

During the summer, cattle should have access to all the lush pasture they can consume. In the winter, depending on your location, free-choice legume hay is best. It should be free from dust, mold, and weeds (Spaulding, 2010).

Fresh water is imperative at all times. Make sure to keep water from freezing in the winter by any means possible (Spaulding, 2010).

Trace minerals and a salt lick are also a good idea. The types of trace minerals needed is all dependent on your location. There are areas that are deficient in or have an overabundance of certain minerals, and it is a lot easier to prevent a deficiency or an overload than to treat it (Spaulding, 2010).

## Calving

In normal birthing's, a calf may be delivered in either a front or a rear presentation; however, most births are front presentation. After the birth, the placenta will be delivered (Spaulding, 2010).

Once the calf has been delivered, clear the nostrils and mouth of mucus and let the mama cow take over. She will clean off her calf and eventually relax to recover. Make sure there are no deep troughs that the calf could fall into and drown (Spaulding, 2010).

Ideally, you should allow a newborn calf to stay with its mother or at least let it nurse from its mother three times daily to get the colostrum milk. After three days, you can begin taking some of the milk for human consumption. Some of the milk still needs to go to the newborn calf (Spaulding, 2010).

## Exercise

Cattle need exercise. This is one of the reasons for an open barn. Without proper movement, the lifespan significantly shortens and can decrease a cow's milk production (Spaulding, 2010).

## Body Temperature

What kind of thermometer should I use? There are two types available. A mercury bulb thermometer is inexpensive but easily broken. There are also electronic thermometers which are a bit more expensive but they last longer and are easier to read (Spaulding, 2010).

The basic thermometers found on the market for humans can do the job with some finagling; however, they do make longer probe thermometers specifically for livestock animals. It is also helpful, but not necessary, to have the disposable plastic sheaths that go over the thermometer so that if any fecal matter gets on the thermometer, its easily removed when the plastic sheath is taken off.

The technique needed to find out our cattle's body temperature is as follows: Stand close to left hand side of the cattle to avoid being kicked. Make sure the cattle know you are there. Lubricate the end of the thermometer with soapy water, lubricant, or soothing salve.  Move the tail to the side (Spaulding, 2010).

If using a mercury thermometer gently shake the mercury down to the bottom of the tube.  Lift the tail and gently insert the thermometer into the cattle's rectum.  Make sure the tip of the thermometer rests against the rectal wall and not into a clump of manure (Spaulding, 2010).

Hold the end of the thermometer tightly to stop it from disappearing up the rectum.  If you are using a mercury thermometer wait at least sixty seconds before removing the thermometer and reading it.  Electronic thermometers will 'beep' when an accurate reading is obtained (Spaulding, 2010).

A precise determination of the normal temperature of cattle does not exist.  Most owners will follow these guidelines (Smaxtec, 2020).
• Calves: 101.3°F to 103.1°F
• Heifers: 100.4°F to 103.1°F
• Adult cattle: 100.94°F to 101.84°F

## Hooves

The hooves of most cattle tend to grow quickly, especially when the animals are pastured on grass and don't get much exercise.  If left untrimmed, the toes often either cross or curl up.  This puts a strain on the tendons.  There are special hoof trimmers for cattle that are used every six months when the animal is standing (Spaulding, 2010).

## Toxic plants to cattle

Plants that are toxic to cattle aren't particularly rare. Take a stroll through any pasture, and there among the grasses you'll find any number of different plants both medicinal and toxic. Small vines, broad-leafed weeds, some wildflowers you might recognize—some you won't. As disquieting as it may be to contemplate, the chances are pretty good that at least some are toxic to cattle. Hundreds of poisonous plants grow in North America, and many are extremely common (Beef, 2019).

The good news, of course, is that the vast majority of those plants pose little threat to cattle. For one thing, most of them are unpalatable, and cattle who are filling up on quality forage aren't likely to spend a lot of time grazing on the few bitter leaves populating their pasture.

Remember how I mentioned that animals have an innate ability to know what plants they need and what plants they do not, also known as Zoopharmacognosy?. Unless your animal is starving, they will most likely avoid toxic plants and just eat plants that are healthy for them.

Another factor that protects cattle is their size. A one-thousand-pound animal has to consume significantly higher quantities of most toxins than a smaller animal does to feel any effects. So, for the most part, as long as your cattle are healthy and your pasture is in good shape, you have little to worry about.

However, some plants are cause for concern either because even a curious nibble can spell doom or because repeated browsing over weeks or months can lead to serious illness and death. This is NOT a complete list; however, this list can help guide you.

Black Walnut (Juglans Nigra)

Black walnut is a tall tree valued for its decorative wood. It grows to be about sixty-five to one hundred feet tall and had a trunk about two to three feet in diameter. The roots of black walnut exude chemicals called juglones that can inhibit the growth of other plants and be toxic to cattle.

Cattle may be affected by black walnut chips or sawdust when they are used for bedding material. Close association with walnut trees while pollen is being shed (typically in May) also produce allergic symptoms in both cattle and humans. The juglone toxin occurs in the leaves, bark and wood of walnut, but these contain lower concentrations than in the roots.


Lupine (Lupinus polyphyllus)

Lupine, also known as bluebonnet, may look like a wildflower, but it is a fast-growing legume in the pea family that just happens to have a tall, showy spire of colorful blooms that are typically purple, but can also be blue, white, or yellow (Mcintosh, 2023).

The greatest risk of lupine for cattle is "crooked calf syndrome" when pregnant cows eat it during a certain part of her pregnancy and the calves are born with cleft palate and skeletal defects.

Other signs of symptoms of lupine poisoning include nervousness, excessive salivation, frothing at the mouth, depression, reluctance to move, lethargy, difficulty breathing, twitching leg muscles, loss of all muscular control, convulsions, coma, and death.

Death Camas (Zigadenus spp)

Death camas is the common name of several species of plants that are poisonous to cattle. The more toxic of these species are grassy death camas (Z. gramineus), meadow death camas (Z. venenosus), foothill death camas (Z. paniculatus), and Nuttall's death camas (Z. nuttallii).

Death camas is one of the first plants to begin growing in the early spring. Without sufficient other forage, death camas may be heavily grazed.

Signs of poisoning include salivation, bloody frothing, nausea, vomiting, muscular weakness, staggering, increase pulse, decreased pulse, labored breathing, gasping, coma, lung congestion, kidney congestion, and death.

Nightshades

Nightshade is a family of plants that includes tomatoes, eggplant, potatoes, and peppers. Tobacco is also in the nightshade family. Nightshades are unique because they contain small amounts of alkaloids. Alkaloids are chemicals that are mainly found in plants. Alkaloids are composed of nitrogen, protects plants from predators, and regulates the plants growth (Zelman, 2023).

If the density of the nightshades is very high, it can potentially poison cattle (Homegrown Herbalist, n.d.)

Signs and symptoms of nightshade poisoning for cattle are labored breathing, expiratory grunting, salivation, nasal discharge, slightly elevated body temperature, drowsiness, progressive weakness, paralysis, trembling, increased heart rate, and gastrointestinal inflammation.

## Poison Hemlock (Conium maculatum)

Poison-hemlock grows throughout the United States and is very toxic to cattle. It has white flowers that grow in small erect clusters and each flower develops into a green, deeply ridged fruit that contains several seeds. It starts growing in the early spring and usually grows for two years, can be six to nine feet tall, and turns grayish brown after maturity.

All parts of poison-hemlock (leaves, stem, fruit, and root) are poisonous. Fresh leaves are unpalatable, so cattle seldom eat hemlock when other feed is available.

Signs that one of your cattle have eaten poison hemlock include ataxia, salivation, lack of coordination, pupil dilation, rapid pulse, weak pulse, respiratory paralysis, coma, nervous trembling, depression, convulsions, gastrointestinal irritation, bloody feces, and death.

## Water Hemlock (Cicuta maculate)

Water hemlock grows in many places in North America. It has small, white flowers that grow in umbrella like clusters, side veins on the leaves, a thick rootstalk, and toxic brown or straw-colored liquid filled stem chambers. The toxic substance is cicutoxin, a highly poisonous unsaturated alcohol that has a strong carrot-like odor. It is found principally in the tubers, but is also present in the leaves and stems during early growth. Leaves and stems lose most of their toxicity as they mature, however green seed heads are poisonous (USDA, n.d.).

It only takes a very small amount of this toxin to kill cattle within hours. It acts directly on the central nervous system to cause violent convulsions, grand mal seizures, and death.

Water hemlock may be confused with poison-hemlock because of the similarity in names however, these two are different plants that cause different types of poisoning.

Signs of poisoning include nervousness, excessive salivation, muscle twitching, pupil dilation, rapid pulse, rapid breathing, tremors, violent convulsions, coma, and death within fifteen minutes.

Larkspur (Delphinium)

Larkspur is a herbaceous plant in the buttercup family. The plants are found throughout the Northern Hemisphere and in certain areas of Africa. It can grow as tall as three feet and have bright blue, pink, yellow, or white flowers on branching stalks (Ehlert, 2022).

Larkspur is palatable to cattle and contain high levels of alkaloids, making them especially toxic. Because of this, larkspur causes the second highest death in livestock from poisonous plants across the western United States. Just five pounds of larkspur consumed within an hour is a lethal dose for a one-thousand-pound cow (Ehlert, 2022).

Signs include nervousness, staggering, salivation, muscular twitching, bloating, respiratory paralysis, and death (Britannica, n.d.).

Buttercups (Ranunculaceae)

There are many different types of buttercup plants. However, the small, yellow buttercups typically found the South are often found in lawns and pastures. They are considered a source of food for bees and hummingbirds although they are considered poisonous and may cause dermatitis (Riccio, 2023).

Normally buttercups are too bitter for livestock but if food is in short supply and many are eaten, blisters on lips and mouths can be seen along with abdominal pain, diarrhea, nervousness, twitching of the ears and lips, labored breathing, partial paralysis, and sometimes convulsions (Riccio, 2023).

Milkweed (Asclepias spp.)

There are several different types of milkweed. Ascelpias Labriformis is the most toxic. Milkweed is a perennial that has greenish-white flowers in umbrella-like clusters with leaves that are narrow or broad. Anything grown above ground is poisonous to cattle (USDA, n.d.)..

Milkweed poisoning occurs frequently in cattle when they do not have enough quality forage to eat. Poisoning may also occur if cattle are fed hay containing large amounts of milkweed (USDA, n.d.).

Signs include depression, weakness, staggered gait, difficulty breathing, pupil dilation, rapid pulse, loss of muscular control, elevated temperature, violent spasms, bloating, respiratory paralysis, and gastroenteritis (USDA, n.d.).

Rhododendron (Rhododendron ponticum)

Rhododendrons are generally large shrubs with leaves that are alternate, simple, leathery, and often evergreen. The flowers are produced in large, showy, terminal clusters, ranging in color from white to purple, to red. The fruits are elongated capsules that split into five sections to release small, scalelike seeds (Colorado State University, n.d.).

All parts of the plant including the nectar is toxic. Most poisoning occurs in the winter months because the leaves are generally evergreen and are attractive to animals when other forages are scarce.  Cattle eating approximately 0.2 percent of their body weight of leaves are likely to develop signs of poisoning (Colorado State University, n.d.).

When cattle ingest rhododendron's, they can show signs of anorexia, excessive salivation, vomiting, colic, and frequent defecation.  They can also show signs of muscle weakness, slow heart rate, paralysis, pneumonia, coma, and death (Colorado State University, n.d.).

Mountain Laurel (Kalmia latifolia)

Mountain-laurel is a broad-leaved evergreen shrub that is ten to thirty feet tall at maturity. The crooked, irregular branches are characteristically contorted, forming dense thickets. The shiny evergreen leaves are simple, alternate, and mostly crowded at the branch tips (Goat World, n.d.).

All parts of mountain laurel are poisonous.  It is possible cattle can survive this poison if they haven't eaten more than 0.2 percent of their body weight.  Those first signs include salivating, vomiting, diarrhea, abdominal pain, and tremors.  Later, they may develop convulsions, coma, and death (Goat World, n.d.).

Black Cherry (Prunus serotina)

Black cherry is a large, native tree found in the Midwest and throughout the eastern United States. The showy white flowers appear as pendulous clusters in early spring, followed by dark, pea-sized fruits in late summer.  The mature bark is dark and scaly, often flipping up on the edges (The Morton Arboretum, n.d.).

If cherry trees are within reach of cattle in the pasture, beware of wilted leaves. Cattle will easily consume these leaves and experience the release of very potent cyanide into the bloodstream. As little as one to four pounds of wilted black cherry leaves could be a lethal dose for a one-thousand-pound dairy cow (PennState Extension, 2023).

Signs of toxicity in cattle can occur within fifteen to twenty minutes following ingestion. These may include salivating, increased respiration, weak pulse, and convulsions. If livestock have collapsed, you may observe kicking or paddling of the legs. Mucus membranes of the animals will be bright red. Livestock will succumb to cyanide poisoning quickly and death will be rapid (PennState Extension, 2023).

Locoweed (Oxytropis)

Locoweed is a perennial with a long tap root. The leaves are eight to twelve inches long with silvery hairs. The white flowers are pea-like with a purple tip on a leafless stalk in a raceme (Colorado State University, n.d.).

Locoweed is poisonous at all times, even when dried. Depending on the duration of locoweed consumption, the poison can be secreted in the milk of lactating cows and will therefore affect the young calves suckling its mother (Colorado State University, n.d.).

Signs of poisoning include congestive heart failure, neurologic issues, and abortions. This poison doesn't kill instantly. It can show in signs of offspring, if the offspring lives, with developmental and growth delays or deformed legs (Colorado State University, n.d.).

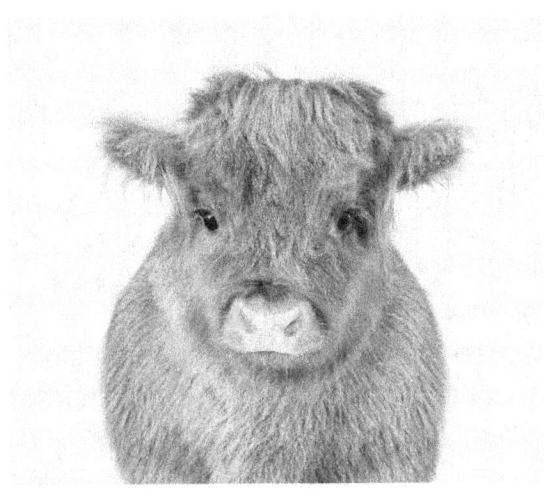

## Chapter 8:

## Cattle Ailments/problems/health concerns

While both dairy and beef cattle are generally quite hardy, it is smart to be aware of health problems that might happen.

Let's take a look at some common cattle health concerns. Any dosing mentioned is based on an adult at one thousand five hundred pounds.

# BLACKLEG

Blackleg is a disease that causes severe losses in cattle from three months to two years of age.

Although blackleg is one of the oldest and most widely recognized causes of death, the way the disease works is still not fully understood. It is believed that cattle ingest the spores which are then absorbed through the intestines and into the bloodstream where they get distributed to multiple tissues, including skeletal and heart muscles. Once there, the white blood cells called "macrophages" engulf them and the organism can survive months to years within these cells without affecting the animal. However, when the oxygen level drops within the muscle cell, for example due to injury and bruising, the spores germinate, and the vegetative bacteria grow and produce the deadly toxin related to tetanus (Adkins, 2021).

These organisms live in the soil for years. They enter cattle's bodies through the digestive tract or through small puncture wounds. Blackleg can appear suddenly and cause death within hours. It gets its name from when skinning the leg of the dead cattle, it appears purple as if they were bruised badly (Spaulding, 2010).

The bacterium produces gas that builds up under the skin of an affected leg, causing the skin to feel similar to "bubble wrap" and makes a crackling, rattling sound known as "crepitation" when pushing the skin down over the affected area. It is also sometimes seen around the neck (Adkins, 2021).

PREVENTION

Veterinarians will always recommend vaccination; however, calves are protected until three to four months of age if they absorbed adequate colostrum from their mothers within a few hours after birth. That milk has bacterial fighting agents which will boost the calf's immune system (NC Cooperative Extension, n.d.).

With calves from three months old and up, I would keep their immune system as high as possible if you chose not to vaccinate.

## TREATMENT

Once blackleg has affected the cattle, not much can be done to treat this condition. In this situation, it is best to keep your affected cattle as comfortable as possible. Give them one cup white willow bark every four hours for pain, along with plenty of water.

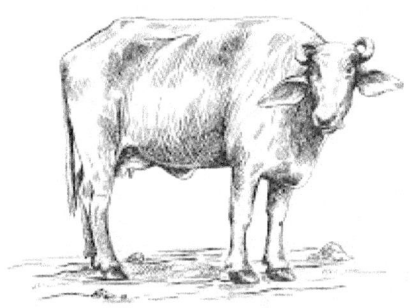

## BLOAT

Bloat is a form of indigestion marked by excessive accumulation of gas in the rumen. Immediately after cattle consume a meal, the digestive process creates gases in the rumen. Most of the gases are eliminated by eructation (belching). Any interruption of this normal gas elimination results in gas accumulation or bloat (Rasby, n.d.).

Bloat can be caused by the amount of roughage being consumed, the rate of roughage intake, the rate of digestion, or it can be an inherited trait (Rasby, n.d.).

Visual signs of bloat in cattle include distension of the left side, discomfort as indicated by stomping of feet or kicking at the belly, labored breathing, frequent urination and defecation, and sudden collapse (Rasby, n.d.).

## PREVENTION

Preventing bloat is desirable not only to reduce deaths but also to reduce the negative effect of bloat on cattle performance (Rasby, n.d.).

Often, proper grazing management can reduce or eliminate bloat problems. Proper grazing management techniques involve providing a consistent and steady diet and controlling access to high bloat-potential plants, especially under moist conditions. When you provide a consistent or gradual change in forage quality and plant species, you maintain uniform rumen conditions and reduce the chance of hungry cattle overeating (Rasby, n.d.).

To prevent bloating, plant mixtures of legume and grass with legumes providing no more than fifty percent of the available forage. Plant non-bloating legumes like birdsfoot trefoil, cicer milkvetch, sainfoin, and lespedeza, or lower-risk legumes like sweet clover and red clover (Ewalt, 1944).

Cascara Sagrada is an herb that you can give to help prevent bloat from happening.  Give three to four tablespoons if you suspect bloating (Karreman, n.d.).


## TREATMENT

It is best to prevent bloat from happening in the first place.  If it does happen, there are some things you can do to help release the gas.  Always make sure there is plenty of fresh water available (Ewalt, 1944).

Movement can sometimes help release some of the gas buildup.  You can also place a three-inch piece of wood in the cattle's mouth as a bit.  This can sometimes stimulate belching (Ewalt, 1944).

Farmers of the past have also had the animal stand with the front feet as high as possible. This alone can help but sometimes they also drench one to two quarts of raw linseed or mineral oil to prevent obstruction of the opening into the rumen and allow excess gas to escape (Ewalt, 1944).

In severe cases, it is possible to insert a tube or hose in the mouth and feed it to the stomach to provide relief.  This doesn't always work, however if it does, large amounts of gas can be released through the tube or by belching (Rasby, n.d.).

As a last resort, use a trocar with canula to puncture the rumen on the left side at the high point half way between the last rib and the hip bone, leaving the canula in the hole to form an opening through which the gas may escape (Ewalt, 1944).

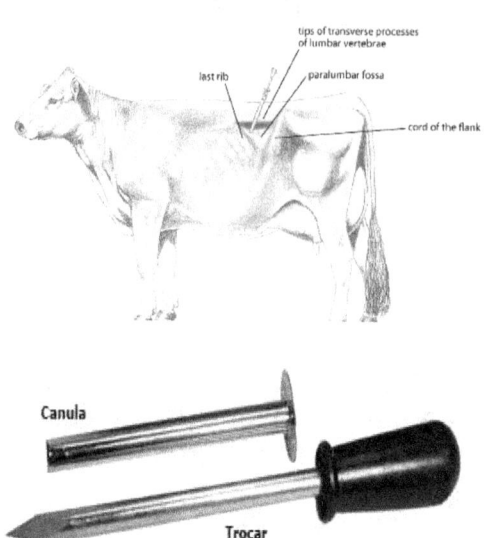

tips of transverse processes
of lumbar vertebrae

last rib

paralumbar fossa

cord of the flank

**Canula**

**Trocar**

## BOVINE VIRUS DIARRHEA

Bovine virus diarrhea, or infectious bovine diarrhea, is a viral disease that is quite common in cattle. It tends to be more of a chronic infection instead of a severe disease (College of Veterinary Medicine, n.d.).

Most animals become exposed through contact with other recently infected or persistently infected (carrier) animals that are shedding the virus. It is also possible for cattle to become infected via contact with contaminated fomites, such as water buckets, calf feeders, feed bunks, IV equipment, nose leads, clothing, people, and cattle trucks (College of Veterinary Medicine, n.d.).

The signs of BVD vary, depending on the immune status of the exposed animals, and the strain of the infecting virus. The incubation period is about three to five days. If susceptible (non-vaccinated) animals are infected with a virulent strain of the virus, the disease will likely appear as an acute, severe sickness, with bloody diarrhea, high fever (105–107 °F), off-feed, mouth ulcers, and often pneumonia. Some infected animals may die, while others will recover, usually within one or two weeks. Occasionally an animal will die very quickly before other signs are apparent. Since BVD is a viral disease, antibiotics are ineffective (College of Veterinary Medicine, n.d.).


## PREVENTION

An effective way to prevent bovine viral diarrhea is boosting your cattle's immune system as much as possible and minimizing exposure of the herd to the virus. You can minimize exposure of the herd by maintaining a closed herd. Since this health concern is commonly associated with new animals entering the herd, maintaining a closed herd is the ideal approach to keep the virus out. If a new animal must be introduced to the herd, isolate cow or steer for two to three weeks in a well-ventilated area. Make sure they are away from the rest of the herd (College of Veterinary Medicine, n.d.).

## TREATMENT

Unfortunately, this is another one of those health concerns in cattle that is untreatable. The best thing to do, if you chose not to vaccinate, is to try to prevent it the best way possible and keep the animal as comfortable as possible (College of Veterinary Medicine, n.d.).

Supportive therapy in the form of lots of fluids and anti-inflammatory and gastro-intestinal herbs may offer some relief to your cattle. Those daily herbs include one cup sage, one fourth cup crushed echinacea root or flower, two to three tablespoons marshmallow root, one fourth cup bentonite clay, one half cup oregano, one half cup ginger, and one tablespoon powdered devil' claw root.

## BROKEN BONE

In cattle, most broken bones occur in the legs and pelvis. Even under the best of conditions, it can happen from a variety of things including trying to step over excessive limbs (Spaulding, 2010).

Signs of a leg break include the animals leg appearing floppy or dangling or if it appears there is a sudden lameness. Signs of a broken pelvis usually is when the steer, cow, or calf can't rise from the ground (Spaulding, 2010).

PREVENTION

To prevent broken bones, be mindful of the cattle's surroundings. Make sure they do not have trees or limbs to fumble over or any sudden drops. Make sure any surface they will stand is safe (Spaulding, 2010).

TREATMENT

The best treatment for a broken leg is to make a splint and treat with herbs. Wrap the leg with a splint and change the herbal poultices frequently. The way the cattle carries its weight along with the cattle's disposition plays a big role with the success. Healing time varies but a broken leg of a steer or cow will usually heal in a couple months (Spaulding, 2010).

A really good herb for broken bones is comfrey. To administer, make a poultice with the comfrey leaves and apply many times a day. In a very short time, the comfrey leaves will penetrate the skin and work on healing the tissue and bone. It is also a good idea to administer this internally as well so it can be healing from the inside out. Forty leaves of comfrey per day in their feed would suffice or making a comfrey herbal tea and adding it to their water bucket or adding fifty drops of a premade tincture into their mouth or water bucket (Homegrown Herbalist, n.d.)

Many of the old western movies will say "shoot a cow with a broken leg". Unless the bone is coming through the skin, more than likely, the animal can be saved (Spaulding, 2010).

With a broken pelvis, it usually occurs as a result of a difficult birth or a bad fall. The steer, cow, or calf will probably not be able to rise from the ground. In this case, you will need to give it time to heal (Spaulding, 2010).

You may need to prop them up using bales of hay or straw. Try to turn them twice a day to prevent pressure sores and to keep circulation in their legs (Spaulding, 2010).

Many with a broken pelvis will lie for a month or more before rising. As long as they are eating, drinking, and appear alert, they have a good chance of eventually getting to their feet. This of course means you will need to bring food, water, and sun shade to the cattle (Spaulding, 2010).

Comfrey is a good herb for a broken pelvis as well, however making a poultice wouldn't work. Giving the comfrey internally would help. You can do this by either feeding forty leaves a day, administering fifty drops three times a day into the mouth or water bucket, or by making an infused tea and adding that to their water bucket (Homegrown Herbalist, n.d.)

## WOUNDS/CUTS

Wounds and/or cuts in cattle are unfortunately extremely common. The most common wounds occur on cattle's limbs and are caused by foreign objects such as fences, gates, farm equipment, and building materials (Rossdales Veterinary Surgeons, n.d.).

There are three main types of wounds: Puncture wounds, lacerations, and abrasions. Abrasions are generally minor wounds that require cleaning and can be treated topically. Lacerations may cause underlying soft tissue damage and infection. Puncture wounds may look small on the surface, but there may be significant damage beneath the skin surface. These may be complicated by infection, as contamination is introduced deep into the wound. Often, the skin heals before the underlying tissue (Rossdales Veterinary Surgeons, n.d.).

PREVENTION

Because cattle wounds occur mostly from fences, gates, farm equipment, and building supplies, it is important for you to make sure such things are out of the cattle's reach and in good repair (Horse Herbs, n.d.)

TREATMENT

With any type of wound, wash it thoroughly with cold water. This will also help reduce any swelling. If the steer or cow is bleeding, use a compaction of the herb called yarrow. Yarrow flowers will stop bleeding (Horse Herbs, n.d.).

The most effective healing herb for a surface wound is comfrey. This is an amazing herb because of the allantoin found in the roots and leaves. Allantoin is a substance that reduces inflammation, helps new skin cells grow, and keeps the skin healthy. Comfrey can be given to cattle internally or topically. If using internally, about forty leaves will help clear any infection inside the cattle and topically, it will help heal the wound very quickly (Horse Herbs, n.d.).

Because comfrey works so well and so quickly at healing, it should never be used on a puncture wound. A puncture wound is very deep and therefore the surface of the skin will heal before the inside layers has a chance to heal. This will cause infection and a lot of issues (Spaulding, 2010).

Manuka honey is also great for wounds. Any honey will work, however specifically manuka honey has healing qualities that can't be beat. Topical use helps to fight infections and speeds recovery (Schell, n.d.).

Calendula is great for cattle skin. It is primarily recognized for its antiseptic, detoxification, and healing properties. It helps prevent the spread of infection, quickens recovery time, combats fevers, and fights infections (Mane Event, n.d.).

With any wound or cut, it is a good idea to use calendula flowers topically and internally. Most cattle will find calendula flowers highly palatable. Dried calendula may be added directly to your cattle's feed or be made into a tea. The tea can be poured over their feed or into their water bucket (Horse Herbs, n.d.).

One other one to mention is cayenne pepper. While cayenne pepper may have a 'kick' at the beginning, using it topically on a cattle's wound can help relieve the pain. When applying, only add a small amount. It will burn for a few seconds so be mindful the cattle may kick and try to get away from it. Once it soaks in, the cattle will find relief (Horse Herbs, n.d.).

Applying a salve or poultice topically of either the comfrey, calendula, manuka honey, or powdered cayenne pepper can be challenging. Depending on where the wound is located on the cattle's body, a dressing can be applied with the salve and/or poultice underneath (Spaulding, 2010).

Ideally the dressing should be applied with firm pressure, but not too tight to restrict blood flow. If it is too loose, it may not stay in place.  The dressing should be changed frequently to reduce inflammation and possible infection (Horse Herbs, n.d.).

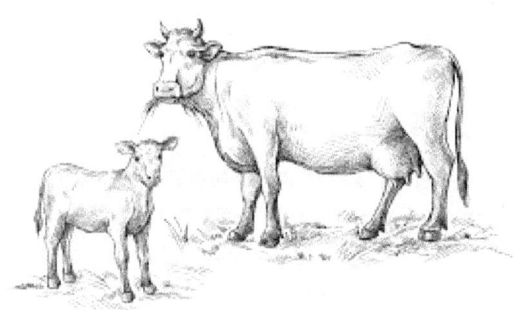

## BITES/STINGS

Bites and stings on your cattle are almost a given. Anything from flies, mosquitos, bees, wasps, spider, etc. will most likely happen. Signs include scratching, biting, and rubbing of the skin, sometimes with loss of hair on the body and tail. Some cattle may be so severely affected that they may have weight loss or show behavioral changes such as restlessness and irritability (Wishgarden, 2018).

## PREVENTION

To help prevent, it is a good idea to have frequent manure removal (it will add up) and eliminating standing water. It may also be a good idea to make sure the bedding is free from any insects that could irritate your cattle (Wishgarden, 2018).

## TREATMENT

There are five herbs that stand out for a bite or sting on cattle. The first one is peppermint. Peppermint oil or crushed leaves are cooling and can soothe itchy or inflamed bites. Simply place a peppermint herbal oil onto the sting or bite and allow to penetrate the area or make a poultice with the crushed leaves and apply a dressing. Change the dressing often (Wishgarden, 2018).

Calendula flower oil or fresh leaves can soothe irritated, itchy skin, and can encourage healthy healing of bites and stings. A simple salve can be created with calendula and beeswax and applied to the wound (Pro Equine Grooms, n.d.).

Witch hazel is an herb that can help relieve minor skin irritations. Create an itch-soothing poultice and apply topically with a dressing that you change frequently. Be careful with witch hazel as the cattle should not eat it in large quantities. Make sure the steer or cow can't reach the dressing with their mouth (Pro Equine Grooms, n.d.).

Comfrey infused oil or fresh juice from leaves can be used topically for bites and stings on cattle. It helps to soothe itching and irritation. Simply apply with a poultice, spray on tincture, or salve (Pro Equine Grooms, n.d.).

And last, but certainly not least, there is plantain. Not to be confuse with the banana leaf, plantain herb is an amazing herb for pulling out the toxins from bee stings or snake bites. It grows almost anywhere and many refer to it as an obnoxious weed. It has a powerful anti-bacterial effect and contains allantoin which is a phytochemical that speeds up wound healing and stimulates the growth of new skin cells. It also helps to stop bleeding, sooth pain, and relieve itching (Pro Equine Grooms, n.d.).

Plantain works best if you can apply a generous amount as soon as the bite or sting happens. It is always best to have a spray-on tincture ready for use, however simply picking the plantain leaves, crushing them in your mouth (mixed with your salvia) can make a spit poultice perfect in a situation where you need to quickly apply a poultice to draw out the poison (Pro Equine Grooms, n.d.).

## FOOT ROT

Foot rot is a highly contagious disease affecting the tissue between the toes of ruminants. It is one of the most common causes of lameness in cattle. Once present in a herd, foot rot can be very difficult to control (Biggs, 2016).

Foot rot is caused by bacteria that effects the connective tissue between the horn and flesh of the hoof and can invade deeper structures of the foot, including joints (Biggs, 2016).

Foot rot tends to be seasonal, with the highest incidence occurring during the wet seasons. Cuts, bruises, puncture wounds, or severe abrasions of the foot due to sharp rocks, sticks, or frozen mud/ice will damage the skin and predispose an animal to foot rot by allowing bacteria to invade and multiply within the tissue (Biggs, 2016).


PREVENTION

The best offense is a good defense. Try to watch out for anything that could harm the cattle's foot and minimize the time they are standing in wet areas. Be very careful of ice and check the animal's feet regularly (Biggs, 2016).

When cattle are moderately to severely deficient in dietary zinc, there may be an increased incidence of foot rot. See zinc in chapter six (Greenpet, n.d.).


TREATMENT

Treatment of foot rot is usually successful, especially when caught early. Treatment should always begin with cleaning and examining the foot. Affected animals should be kept in dry areas until healed, if possible (Greenpet, n.d.).

Herbs can be used, but it is highly recommended to use them both internally and externally. Internally via tincture, tea, or by eating fresh herbs. Externally via tincture, salve, or herbal oil. If giving fresh herbs, five to ten cloves (depending on weight) of garlic internally per day is recommended as an antibiotic. White willow bark can help with pain and is gentle on the stomach. It contains salicin which helps reduce body temperature. A steer or cow can have one-fourth cup powdered white willow bark twice daily as an anti-inflammatory, and one tablespoon powdered devil's claw root twice daily as an anti-inflammatory (Greenpet, n.d.).

**FOOTROT**

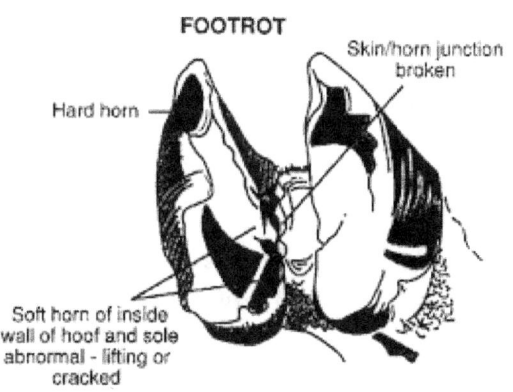

Skin/horn junction broken

Hard horn

Soft horn of inside wall of hoof and sole abnormal - lifting or cracked

## INFECTIOUS BOVINE RHINOTRACHEITIS

Infectious bovine rhinotracheitis is an infectious virus caused by the bovine herpesvirus. Symptoms include respiratory distress, abortion, red and swollen eyes, weakness, lack of appetite, and very inflamed mucous membranes of the nose (Spaulding, 2010).

A fever up to 108 degrees Fahrenheit is also a symptom. A cow with a genital infection may show a raised tall head, increased urination, a swollen viva, ulcers of the vulva, a vaginal discharge, or pustules on the vulva (Spaulding, 2010).

Affected cattle will usually recover in a couple weeks, but they remain contagious to other cattle for several weeks (Spaulding, 2010).


PREVENTION

Because this virus is spread between cattle, it is best to keep any newly introduced cattle isolated in a quarantined area away from your herd. If you do this for eight to ten weeks, you can make sure there is no transmission to your already established herd (Spaulding, 2010).


TREATMENT

Of course, there are modern vaccines available but to avoid these, good herbal routes are to use herbs to increase the immune system and use herbs to knock out any secondary bacterial infections, which are common (Spaulding, 2010).

Daily herbs that may help internally with the bacterial infections include one cup calendula flowers, four tablespoons echinacea flower spread out through the day, five to ten garlic cloves, a big handful of dandelion leaf, and a big handful of chaparral leaves.  It is also a good idea to have them consume yarrow.  Yarrow is an excellent fever reducer; however, large quantities can be toxic to cattle.  Simply give one teaspoon powdered yarrow flower daily.

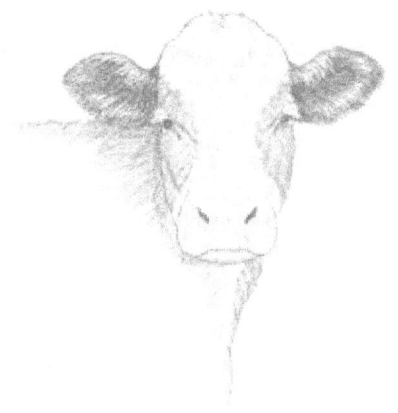

## JOHNE'S DISEASE

Johne's disease is a contagious and chronic, infection that affects primarily the small intestine of ruminants. If not caught soon enough, fatality is high. It spreads through the manure of affected animals, often contaminating the pasture, water, and feed. Even a calf can contract this infection after nursing from its mother's dirty udder (Spaulding, 2010).

Symptoms include diarrhea with a foul odor, fatigue, and weight loss. Fever is not usually seen in cattle with this disease. Although humans cannot contract Johne's disease, it is much like crohn's disease in humans (Spaulding, 2010).

Unfortunately, the inflammation thickens the intestinal wall of cattle and prevents nutrients from being absorbed, leading to extreme weakness and eventually, death (USDA, n.d.).

## PREVENTION

Good management and hygiene of maternity areas, clean feed, clean feed delivery systems, and clean water are basic ways to prevent Johne's disease (College of Veterinary Medicine, 2021).

## TREATMENT

In western medicine, there is no cure for this long-lasting and chronic disease of the intestines. Prevention is the best route; however, there has been promising research on this topic recently showing how cattle with this disease have a very low vitamin D level. Therefore, if you increase the vitamin D, logic is that it will help your herd (USDA, n.d.).

Green leafy vegetables like four cups daily of swiss chard and one cup daily of spinach are good sources of vitamin E for cattle. High vitamin E herbs include a half cup oregano daily and two to three whole cayenne pepper or one tablespoon cayenne pepper powder daily (Nickel, 2020).

I would also suggest having the cattle's immune system in tip top shape with proper diet and herbal supplementation.

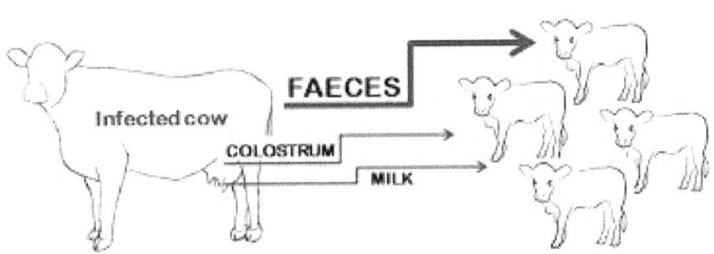

## LEPTOSPIROSIS

Leptospirosis is a contagious bacterial disease in cattle and humans. It is spread through contact with streams, ponds, or surface water contaminated with feces or urine of affected animals (Spaulding, 2010).

Symptoms include fever, weakness, anemia, abortion, and lowered/abnormal milk production. There may be blood in the urine (Spaulding, 2010.)


PREVENTION

The best way to stop this bacterial disease is to keep new incoming cattle away from the other herd for three to four weeks. Also, keep cattle away from ponds or streams with fencing and keep any feed free of rodent contamination (Spaulding, 2010).


TREATMENT

For daily treatment at the first signs of Leptospirosis, use one-fourth cup turmeric, one-half cup ginger, one tablespoon powdered cayenne pepper, five whole onions, and four cups oregano leaves (Price, 2017).

## LICE/MANGE

Lice can appear on cattle at any time of the year but they usually become a problem in the colder months when there is less daylight during the days (Spaulding, 2010).

The first signs of lice you usually notice is when the cattle begin rubbing and scratching themselves on fences or the barn. Sometimes, they will look like they have dandruff or parts of their hair, especially around the neck, will wear off their skin (Spaulding, 2010).

Lice are very small, oval-shaped critters. Their tiny head sometimes will have a reddish tint. If there are a significant number of lice on cattle, they can cause anemia and/or bleed the animals to death (Spaulding, 2010).

Mange is the term used to describe a mite infection and the damage they do on the cattle's skin. They can leave moth-eaten appearances on the skin, scales, crusty spots, pustules, and thickened skin (The Cattle Site, 2022).


PREVENTION

Because lice do not like the sunlight, it is best to keep the cattle outside away from the barn as much as possible for a couple weeks. This will allow you to come in with food grade diatomaceous earth and sprinkle over the bedding or inside areas. This should naturally kill off the lice (OACC, 2009).

TREATMENT

Complete isolation is a must for an animal with mange (Spaulding, 2010). If you notice your cattle do have lice, put diatomaceous earth on them. If you still notice they are there after a couple days, rub a light coat of linseed oil all over the animal's body or you can use neem oil. Repeat after one week to control any newly hatched lice (OACC, 2009).

When purchasing neem oil, you must make sure you have the correct type. Neem oil comes from the Neem tree which is native to India and South Asia. Azadirachta is a chemical substance found in the seeds of the neem tree. The neem oil you purchase must be cold pressed with Azadirachta included in the ingredient list. The neem oil you purchase in many retail stores do not contain Azadirachta. The makers of some neem oil will extract neem from the leaves with heat which does make a neem substance, but not necessarily what will kill mites (WebMD, n.d.).

You can also use wild bergamot (Monarda fistulosa), AKA bee balm, topically as a salve or herbal oil on the animal. Black walnut hulls and calendula flower is also very effective when used topically as a salve or herbal oil. As for internal use, one cup of calendula flowers and five to ten cloves of garlic can be given daily (Homegrown Herbalist, n.d.).

## MASTITIS

Mastitis is an inflammation of a cow's mammary glands. Each situation is different, but most cattle exhibit an udder that looks very clogged and swollen. It can have a watery or bloody discharge. Keep in mind that some cows' udders will swell a bit and feel harder than normal to the touch a few days to a week after freshening. It is a good idea to keep a watch on her body temperature for the first week after giving birth (Spaulding, 2010).

There are three different types of mastitis: Acute, Gangrene, and Chronic. Acute mastitis develops rapidly and is often brought on by stress. Usually there is a marked reduction in milk production, flecks or gummy strings in the milk. The udder is usually hot and swollen in one or more quarters. Their body temperature is also usually high, she acts sick, and she usually will come off of feed (Spaulding, 2010).

Gangrene Mastitis can follow acute mastitis or develop suddenly on its own. A cold udder is not a good sign. It often means the blood supply has died and the teat will literally rot off if the cow doesn't die first (Spaulding, 2010).

With chronic mastitis, the same cow or cows will show repeated periodic flare-ups of mastitis. A cow with chronic mastitis will show little to no signs of being sick. The mastitis lies hidden in scar tissue and any stress lets it break out again (Spaulding, 2010).

PREVENTION

Mastitis is by far easier to prevent than to treat. This is the case with many diseases. Start by eliminating trouble areas such as high concrete steps into the barn. Unfortunately, cows will hang their udders on high steps like this which can cause bacteria to enter the teat. Also, if possible, keep cows from lying in muddy areas, where they can chill their udders in cold weather and pick up bacteria at the same time (Spaulding, 2010).

When a cow has had a calf or calves, it is best to hand milk all four udders several times a day. Don't do this until after the third day after delivery, as the calves will need the colostrum in the milk. Humans should not drink the milk from an udder in which mastitis is suspected. Massage the udders with a warm herbal salve of calendula flowers, plantain, and echinacea. This will help soothe the inflamed mammary glands. Milking the udder with mastitis will help flush out the causative bacteria. If you have more than one cow to milk, it is best to hand milk the one with mastitis last as to not infect the other cows (Spaulding, 2010).

Always dip their teats after milking. This helps prevent mastitis and also chapping (another stress). Also keep the hair around the teats clipped back. Hair encourages the clinging of filth and makes it impossible to wash the udder thoroughly (Spaulding, 2010).

TREATMENT

For internal use, a mixture of one or more of the following herbs will be beneficial daily. One fourth cup of echinacea root or flower, five to ten cloves of garlic, four big handfuls of olive leaves, two tablespoons pau d-arch tree bark, four big handfuls of red clover flowers, 4 tablespoons powdered rose hips, 1 powdered teaspoon of Siberian ginseng root (taken in the morning and with food), and one cup calendula flowers (Spaulding, 2010).

For topical use, make a warm tea with comfrey leaves, comfrey roots, and calendula flowers and dip the udders into it. After the tea temperature has decreased, use a salve made from the same as the tea which will adhere to the udders and give relief through the night (Spaulding, 2010).

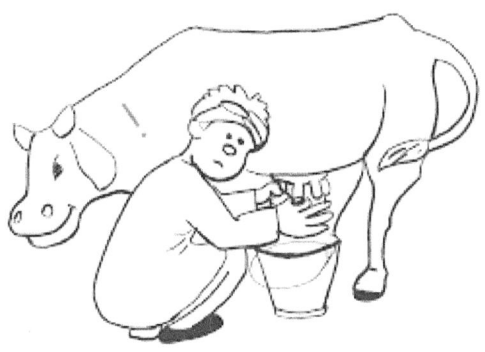

## MILK FEVER

To an inexperienced person, milk fever would indicate 'fever'. However, milk fever does not mean the animal has a fever. Milk fever occurs in high producing milk cows, usually Jersey cows, and is often in cows that have had two or more calves (Spaulding, 2010).

Milk fever can be seen several days before calving and is caused by low blood calcium. It causes paralysis in all cases. In some cows, a characteristic bend, or kink, in their neck is seen in which they are unable to hold straight (Spaulding, 2010).

PREVENTION

Cut down on grain and don't milk out a cow completely for the first 3 days following freshening (VCA, n.d.).

Replace alfalfa, which is very high in calcium and potassium, with grass-based hay as their diet a few days before freshening. This may sound contradicting, especially since milk fever is caused by low calcium levels; however, the high levels of potassium that alfalfa contains, diminishes the much-needed calcium (VCA, n.d.).

Herbs high in calcium that can be fed to your cow are two cups of chamomile flower daily (Plant Archives, 2019) and four cups of dried stinging nettle daily. If you allow the stinging nettle to dry for a couple days, the stinging part of the nettle isn't as bad and the cows are more likely to eat it (Research Gate, 2010).

Plantain is also high in calcium. Twelve to fifteen cups of plantain daily is good for your cow. It grows almost everywhere so obtaining this amount wouldn't be difficult. To raise the calcium levels, I would also suggest having a daily bale of oat straw, all the dandelion leaves, flowers, and roots that she can eat daily, and five cups of dried basil daily (Mendicino, 2023).

## TREATMENT

In modern veterinary medicine, an injection of calcium may be given. This can have harmful side effects because it is a powerful stimulant to the heart when given in large doses at one time. If the cow has heart abnormalities, this can kill her. It is best to prevent this in the first place by feeding her the herbs listed above. If this still happens, begin feeding her the above herbs and keep her well hydrated (Mendicino, 2023).

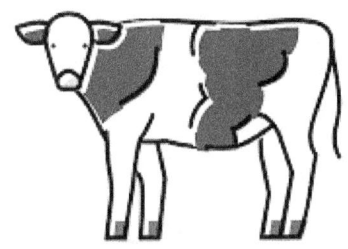

## PINKEYE

Pinkeye is also known as infectious keratitis.  Pink eye is a highly contagious disease that impacts productivity and is incredibly painful to cattle (Ralco, 2022).  It is most common during the summer months.  Usually, the first sign of pinkeye is an eye that is tearing followed by squinting and appear bloodshot.  If left untreated, sometimes it can clear up on its own but generally, a bluish, cloudy film may appear over the entire eye.  Eyesight will be lost in that eye (Spaulding, 2010).

Pinkeye is spread by flies that walk on the tears of the infected eyes and then move on to other animals (Spaulding, 2010).


## PREVENTION

Fly control during the summer will help prevent pinkeye in your cattle.  Also, feeding five to ten garlic cloves daily will help ward off the flies (Ralco, 2022).


## TREATMENT

If possible, confine any cattle showing symptoms of pink eye so as to prevent the spread throughout the heard. It is important to protect the eyes from sunlight so keep them in the barn away from other animals with plenty of feed and water. Dab raw honey and aloe vera juice directly to the eyeball to help treat this condition (PCO, 2020).

## PNEUMONIA

Pneumonia, also known as bovine respiratory disease, is inflammation of the lung tissues and airways. It usually affects calves and is brought on by stress such as changes in weather, shipping, changes in feed, or confinement in damp areas (AHDB, n.d.).

There are two types of cattle pneumonia: Acute and chronic. Symptoms of acute pneumonia include reduction in feeding, dull demeanor, dropping of the head, increased respiratory rate, nasal discharge, cough, and raised temperature that could lead to death. The onset of chronic pneumonia is more gradual with no distinct ill phase. The animal may appear to still eat well but may have a slight nasal discharge. Sometimes chronic pneumonia symptoms may be a cough with an increased respiratory rate (AHDB, n.d.).

PREVENTION

The best way to prevent pneumonia is to avoid moving the cattle in extreme outdoor conditions (heat, cold, or very dusty), avoid overcrowding with grazing and transportation, avoid sudden diet changes, and avoid mixing of different herds. Provide appropriate shelter, ensure continual access to clean water, and separate any affected animals from the non-infected (MLA, n.d.).

TREATMENT

If pneumonia is suspected, isolate any affected animals in a well-ventilated area protected from excessive cold or heat. Make sure to maintain hydration and provide easy access to water and feed. It is important to keep physical stress to a minimum (MLA, n.d.).

I would suggest getting good respiratory herbs and immune system herbs daily into the cattle. Good herbs for the respiratory system include a big handful of Chaparral leaves and three to four grape leaves (Homegrown Herbalist, n.d.).

Good herbs for the Immune system daily include one fourth cup crushed echinacea root or flower, five to ten cloves of garlic, four big handfuls of olive leaf, four big handfuls of red clover flower, four tablespoons powdered rose hips, and one powdered teaspoon of siberian ginseng root (Homegrown Herbalist, n.d.).

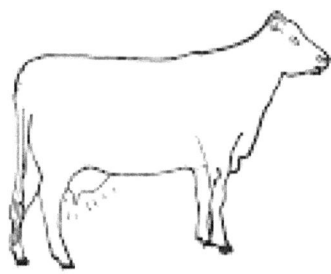

## RINGWORM

Ringworm is a rash caused by a fungal infection. Most people think this is a worm or caused by a worm but it is not. It is a dermatitis caused by a fungus that usually appears on the face or neck as rough, scaly, patches of baldness (Spaulding, 2010).

Ringworm is very contagious and is most often seen in the winter months. It thrives in long hair and dark conditions. Small patches of ringworm are not dangerous, but if not treated, they can spread over quite a large portion of the body. This interferes with normal skin functions. Having ringworm is a stress on their body and can cause your cattle to be more prone to other health problems (Spaulding, 2010).

## PREVENTION

Cleaning and disinfecting barns does a good job. Cleaning halters and grooming equipment should also be cleaned well.

## TREATMENT

To treat ringworm, remove the thick, scaly dandruff by soaking with warm, soapy water (Spaulding, 2010). Apply either an herbal oil or herbal salve made with bergamot (Monarda fistulosa), black walnut hulls, calendula flower, chamomile flower, and goldenseal root several times a day (Homegrown Herbalist, n.d.). Make sure to apply the herbal oil or salve from the outside and work your way inward. Scrubbing from the inside out can spread the lesions. Topical iodine tinctures and getting the cattle into sunlight has also been shown to be effective. It may also be a good idea to give the animal five to ten garlic cloves a day to fight the infection from inside (Spaulding, 2010).

If an herbal oil or salve cannot be applied several times a day, spraying a tea with the previous herbs may be an option or spraying a tincture onto the areas several times a day.

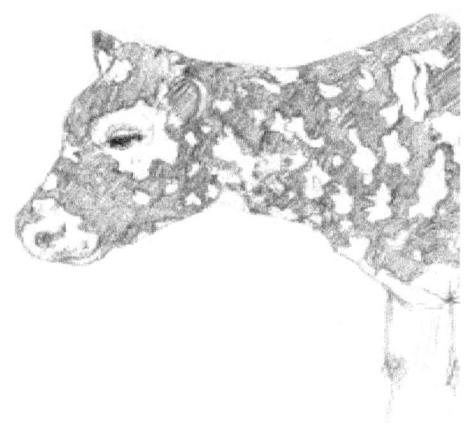

## SCOURS/DIARRHEA

Scours is a term used for diarrhea in farm animals. It can affect both young and older animals. Calves, up to around a month old, are usually the ones who suffer the most. The most common causes are stress and overeating, especially over consumption of milk (Spaulding, 2010).

In young calves, the feces are typically yellowish and a bit gooey but still has form to it. If it is scours, you will see puddles of mush in their bedding instead of manure or wet manure stuck to their tail. Unfortunately, if not treated quickly enough, a calf can die, even if it seems in good spirits (Spaulding, 2010).

In adult cattle, when they are on lush pasture in the summer months, sometimes their stools can become quite loose. If in doubt, bring the animal into the barn or into a dry lot and feed it hay for a day or two. If the stool returns to normal, you know it isn't diarrhea (Spaulding, 2010).

In the winter months when cattle are sometimes confined in a barn, they can become susceptible to 'winter scours' or also known as winter dysentery. This comes on suddenly but rarely kills cattle (Spaulding, 2010).


PREVENTING

For calves, if you notice the stools are slightly loose, cut the milk feedings in half. Make sure they have adequate water to make up for the liquid they are not receiving with the milk (Spaulding, 2010).

In adult cattle, ensuring that cattle are in good health with a high immune system reduces their susceptibility to becoming infected while examination and quarantine practices are good ways to make sure you are not introducing unwell cattle into your herd (Agriculture and Food, n.d.).


## TREATMENT

Mix a half pound of barley in one gallon of warm water and make a barley tea. Let this simmer for an hour. Strain the barley out and once it is room temperature, feed one pint at a time, every two hours throughout the day. If for a calf, feed this in place of milk (Spaulding, 2010).

One cup of calendula flowers daily, one cup common sage daily, one fourth cup powdered echinacea root or flower daily, five to ten cloves garlic cloves daily, five cc's Angellica seed tincture two to four times daily, two to three tablespoons marshmallow root daily, one fourth cup of bentonite clay daily, a big handful of chaparral leaves daily, and two cups of chamomile flowers daily are great herbs to help diarrhea in cattle (Homegrown Herbalist, n.d.).

## TEAT AND UDDER INJURIES

Because of cow's weight and clumsiness, cows have more udder and teat injuries than any other domestic animal. The ways they can get injured are getting stepped on, snagged, scaped, punctured, bitten, etc. Milk veins are also at a greater risk of injury. They can be three inches across, making it a prime target for injury (Midgette, 2023).

## PREVENTION

Be aware of objects that her udder and teats could rub against. Often times, there may be a step down into a barn and a cow will injure her teats this way. Also, make sure other cattle with her are not crowded. The chances of her udder being stepped on is higher when she doesn't have a lot of room to move around (Midgette, 2023).

## TREATMENT

If a bleeding wound does occur on the udder or teat, put a clean cloth on her injury and hold it tight while someone else gets yarrow flowers. Pack the yarrow flowers around the area and the bleeding should stop. Once the bleeding has stopped and there are no signs of more bleeding returning, use a powdered poultice on the area. This poultice should consist of Comfrey root, Calendula, Plantain, and Marshmallow Root. The cow will need to stay away from other cattle until healed. After a few days of the poultice, and reapplying often, switch to an herbal oil or salve made from the same poultice powder. Reapply often until healed. If she is in milk, it is best to milk her, but do not drink any of the milk until she has healed (Spaulding, 2010).

Can you identify these herbs?

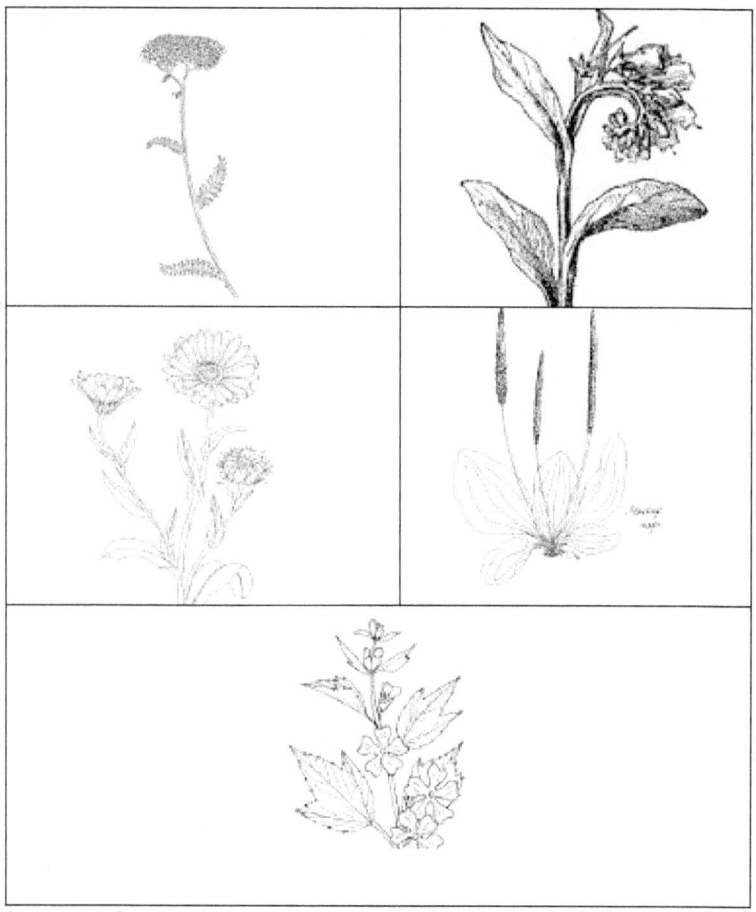

Answer (top left to right):  Yarrow, Comfrey, Calendula, Plantain, and Marshmallow.

## TETANUS

Tetanus is a serious infectious disease of the central nervous system. Tetanus often occurs in cattle with a puncture wound or castration (Midgette, 2023).

A cow or calf with tetanus will usually be reluctant to move. Sometimes the symptoms of tetanus mimic rabies. These symptoms include standing with its neck stretched out, drooling, and being unable to eat or drink. The membrane in the corner of their eyes typically covers nearly half of the eyeball and they will become more and more stiff (Spaulding, 2010).

## PREVENTION

Make sure that any surgical procedures are done in a very clean and sterile environment and also make sure nails are properly secured in the barn. Sometimes they will snag themselves on nails that have begun to pop out (The Cattle Site, 2022).

## TREATMENT

Many of the herbs available for tetanus do not grow in the United States. These are herbs in which it is a good idea to stock up on. Freeze dry them or preserve them so that you have them if you need them. For an adult, (smaller dose for calves), mix together one part Rhizoma Arisaematis, one part Rhizoma Gastrodiae, one part Radix Saposhnikoviae, two parts Fructus Xanthii, and two and a half parts Cortex Jujubae.

## PARASITES (WORMS)

The most common types of worms in cattle are tapeworms, roundworms, and flukes. Some of these are microscopic and cannot be seen with the naked eye. Signs of worm infestation include weight loss, potbelly, bad hair coat, general weakness, and coughing.

It is important to know the type of worms the cattle have in order to treat accordingly. An easy way to do this is to send a fecal sample to your veterinarian. If you do not have access to a veterinarian, it is possible to do a fecal analysis on your own; however, you will need the proper equipment including a microscope, slides, and fecal floatation solution.

Do not deworm your cattle without knowing what type of worms they have. All wormers do not get rid of all worms. On top of that, if you suspect worms and they do not have worms, a commercial dewormer can kill them (Te Pari, n.d.).

PREVENTION

The best way to prevent worms in your cattle is to not allow the cattle to overgraze pastures. You should also make sure their manure is spread out on hot days in order to kill worm eggs and larvae that may be in the feces, and to rotate your cattle often. Having a lot of land will allow you to do this. You can also feed worming herbs regularly to prevent any parasites from forming. For prevention, herbs that can be given include five garlic cloves, a handful of wormwood leaf, and a handful of mugwort leaves.

TREATMENT

The best way to treat parasites herbally in cattle is through a mixture of herbs. This can be given fresh, as a tea, or as a tincture. Combine two tablespoons black walnut hulls, one tablespoon Cascara Sagrada root, two garlic cloves, two tablespoons marshmallow root, two tablespoons Oregon grape root, two tablespoons psyllium, two tablespoons wormwood leaf, and two tablespoons mugwort leaf. Feed this to each cattle two times a day for two weeks as treatment.

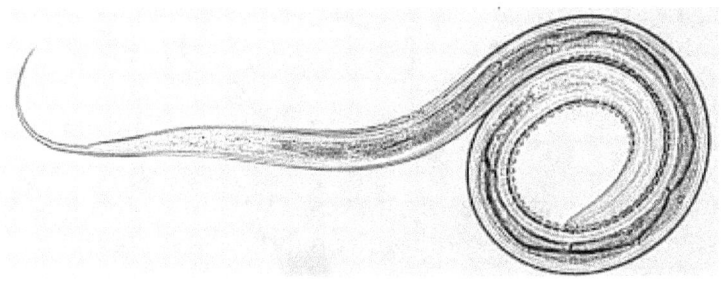

## SHIPPING FEVER

Shipping fever, also known as hemorrhagic septicemia or transit fever, is an acute respiratory disease that occurs in cattle who go through a major stress. It is often brought on when cattle are shipped, however it can happen without being shipped. Being shipped is merely a major stress to them (Spaulding, 2010).

An affected animal often has a high temperature with rapid breathing and a raspy cough. There may be a heavy nasal discharge along with diarrhea. If the lungs are filled with fluid and pus or dehydration occurs, the animal can die. They can be highly contagious to other animals (Spaulding, 2010).

PREVENTION

Isolate any new cattle away from your normal herd for at least two weeks. Provide adequate ventilation and clean barn areas (ProEarth, n.d.).

If you know your steer, cow, or calf will be going through a stressful event soon, give your animal a diet high in roughage. This may reduce the incidence of shipping fever (ProEarch, n.d.).

TREATMENT

A combination of one or all of these herbs can be beneficial for shipping fever.

Usnea (Tincture)

    Adult: Twenty drops three times a day.

Calf: Ten drops three times a day.

Usnea (Powdered)

Adult:  Two teaspoons two times a day.

Calf:  Just a little over a half teaspoon two times a day.

_____

Thyme (Tincture)

Adult:  Twenty drops three times a day.

Calf:  Ten drops three times a day.

Thyme (Powdered)

Adult:  One tablespoon three to four times a day.

Calf:  One half tablespoon three times a day.

_____

Eucalyptus leaves (Powdered)

Adult: One tablespoon three to four times a day.

Calf:  One half tablespoon three times a day.

Eucalyptus (Dried leaves)

Adult:  Just over a half teaspoon two times a day.

Calf:  One third of a teaspoon, split.  One in morning, one in evening.

_____

White Horehound (Powdered)

Adult: Five to eight tablespoons once per day.

Calf: One heaping tablespoon to five tablespoons once per day.

---

Bloodroot (Tincture)

Adult: Five to six drops two times a day.

Calf: Three drops two times a day.

---

Mullein Root (Powdered)

Adult: One heaping **tablespoon** twice a day.

Calf: One half heaping teaspoon twice a day.

Lobelia (Inflata, L.) (Tincture)

Adult: Two tablespoons twice a day.

Calf: Just a little less than one teaspoon

twice a day.

(NODPA, n.d.).

If you have enjoyed this book, this information, along with nine other animals, will be available in "Herbal Animal Care for the Homesteader" which will be available on Amazon, Books-A-Million, Barnes and Noble, and many other popular bookstores soon. I appreciate the purchase of this book. I wish nothing but the best health for your cattle!

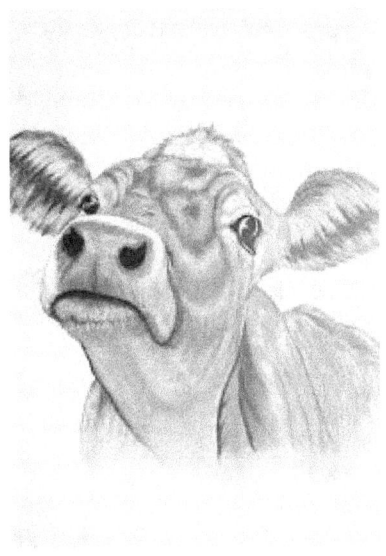

# References for Cattle:

ACKO (2023, December 11). *Overview of zinc and ayurvedic medicine.* https://www.acko.com/health-insurance/zinc-ayurvedic-medicine/

Adkins, T.J. (2021, September 11). *10 Frequently asked questions about blackleg.* https://www.somerset-kentucky.com/news/lifestyles/10-frequently-asked-questions-about-blackleg/article_d26c814f-38e2-5419-9e0d-87014826c4a9.html#:~:text=Flooding%20may%20spread%20the%20spores,throughout%20the%20year%20in%20Kentucky.

Agriculture and Food (2019, September 3). *Cobalt deficiency in sheep and cattle.* https://www.agric.wa.gov.au/livestock-biosecurity/cobalt-deficiency-sheep-and-cattle#:~:text=All%20ruminants%20(including%20sheep%2C%20cattle,vitamin%20B12%20deficiency%20in%20livestock.

Agriculture and Food (2019, November 25). *Selenium deficiency in cattle.* https://www.agric.wa.gov.au/feeding-nutrition/selenium-deficiency-cattle

AHV (n.d.). *What causes calcium deficiency?* https://ahvint.com/us/dairy-cows-calves/calcium-deficiency-has-major-impact-on-herd-health/#:~:text=A%20cow%20that%20has%20a,get%20up%20properly%2C%20for%20example.

Alberta (n.d.). *Vitamin E requirements in cow and finishing beef rations.* https://www.alberta.ca/vitamin-e-requirements-in-cow-and-finishing-beef#:~:text=Vitamin%20E%20is%20a%20fat,muscular%20dystrophy%20in%20young%20calves.

All Animals (2021, July 4). *Can cows eat pumpkin leaves?* https://allanimalsfaq.com/cow/can-cows-eat-pumpkin-leaves/

Animal Welfare Institute (n.d.). *Cattle.* https://awionline.org/content/cattle

Apelian, N. (2021). *The Lost Book of Herbal Remedies.* pp. 33-42

Baily, E. (2017). *Vitamins for beef cattle.* https://extension.missouri.edu/publications/g2058#:~:text=Under%20normal%20conditions%2C%20cattle%20receive,of%20sun%2Dcured%20forages%20daily.

Beef (2019, May 15). *Fact Sheet: Poisonous Plants for Cattle.* https://www.beefmagazine.com/pasture/fact-sheet-poisonous-plants-for-cattle

Beef Cattle (2019, September 3). *Can beef cattle suffer from thiamine deficiency and if so what are the causes and effects?* https://beef-cattle.extension.org/can-beef-cattle-suffer-from-thiamine-deficiency-and-if-so-what-are-the-causes-and-effects/

Better Crops (1998). *Potassium in Animal Nutrition.* http://www.ipni.net/publication/bettercrops.nsf/0/9C7E99D11D5EE7758525798000820369/%24FILE/Better%20Crops%201998-3%20p32.pdf

Block, E. (2013, April 10). *Make sure cows get enough early lactation potassium.* https://www.agproud.com/articles/23451-make-sure-cows-get-enough-early-lactation-potassium#:~:text=Dietary%20potassium%20is%20a%20significant,function%20and%20cow%20well%2Dbeing.

Brittanica (2023, December 19). *Cattle.* https://www.britannica.com/animal/cattle-livestock

Britannica (n.d.). Larkspur. https://www.britannica.com/plant/larkspur-plant

Coates, J. (2012, October 25). *The History and Use of Herbal Medicine and its Use Today with Pets.* https://www.petmd.com/blogs/fullyvetted/2012/oct/history_and_use_of_herbal_medicine_and_use_in_pets-29279

College of Veterinary Medicine (n.d.). *Bovine Viral Diarrhea.* https://www.vet.cornell.edu/animal-health-diagnostic-center/programs/nyschap/modules-documents/bovine-viral-diarrhea-background-management-and-control#:~:text=What%20is%20Bovine%20Viral%20Diarrhea,be%20a%20serious%2C%20costly%20disease.

College of Veterinary Medicine (2001, August 14). *Principles of Johne's Prevention and Control.* https://www.vet.cornell.edu/animal-health-diagnostic-center/programs/nyschap/modules-documents/Johnes-Principles#:~:text=Good%20management%20and%20hygiene%20of,parasites%20spread%20by%20fecal%20shedding.

Colorado State University (n.d.). Locoweed, white point-locoweed, crazy weed. https://poisonousplants.cvmbs.colostate.edu/plant/12

Colorado State University (n.d.). *Rhododendrone.* https://poisonousplants.cvmbs.colostate.edu/plant/111

Cooke, R.P. (2015, August 3). *Cooling cattle off.* https://www.farmprogress.com/corn/cooling-cattle-off

Da Silva, D. (2019, September 27). *The role of calcium in transition cows.* https://formafeed.com/the-role-of-calcium-in-transition-cows/#:~:text=It%20is%20essential%20for%20muscle,cannot%20be%20g ained%20back%20later.

Duffy, R. (2023, September). *A review of the impact of dietary zinc on livestock health.* https://www.sciencedirect.com/science/article/pii/S2773050623000381#:~:t ext=Zinc%20deficiency%20can%20lead%20to,and%20increased%20susc eptibility%20to%20diseases.

Ehlert, K. (2022, October 24). *Poisonous Plants on Ranchlands : Larkspur and Poisonvetch.* https://extension.sdstate.edu/poisonous-plants-rangelands-larkspur-and-poisonvetch#:~:text=Five%20pounds%20of%20larkspur%20consumed,les s%20susceptible%20to%20larkspur%20poisoning.

Ewalt, H.P. (1944, August). *Bloat in Cattle.* file:///C:/Users/Apbru/Downloads/ECNO436%20(2).pdf

Farm Health (n.d.). *Milk Fever in Cattle.* https://www.farmhealthonline.com/US/disease-management/cattle-diseases/milk-fever/

Feek, R. (2023). *'Why We Homestead', The Homesteading Guide.* pp. 7-11.

FitAudit (n.d.). *Phosphorus in herbs.* https://fitaudit.com/categories/lvs/phosphorus

Goat World (n.d.). *Mountain Laurel.* https://www.goatworld.com/health/plants/mountainlaurel.shtml

Groot, M. (n.d.). *Natural Dairy Cow Health.* https://edepot.wur.nl/194289

Karreman, Hue (n.d.). *Preventing pasture bloat.* https://www.ecofarmingdaily.com/raise-healthy-livestock/cattle/preventing-pasture-bloat/#:~:text=Herbal%20laxatives%20like%20Cascara%20sagrada,chokin g%20off%20the%20animal%20internally.

Lalman, D. (2017, March). *Vitamin and Mineral Nutrition of Grazing Cattle.* https://extension.okstate.edu/fact-sheets/vitamin-and-mineral-nutrition-of-grazing-cattle.html

Mcintosh, J. (2023, July 30). *How To Grow and Care for Lupine.* https://www.thespruce.com/growing-lupine-flowers-1316034

McKinnon, J. (2014, February 19). *Supplementing vitamins A, D, and E to beef cattle.* https://www.canadiancattlemen.ca/nutrition/supplementing-vitamins-a-d-and-e-to-beef-cattle/

Medicino, S. (2023, February 22). *5 herbs high in vitamin d.* https://botanicalinstitute.org/herbs-high-in-vitamin-d/

Mendicino, S. (2023, April 3). *6 Herbs High in Calcium.* https://botanicalinstitute.org/herbs-high-in-calcium/

Midgette, B. (2023, August 22). *Ugly Udderness.* Pg 82-27.

MLA (n.d.). *Why do cattle need phosphorus?* https://www.mla.com.au/globalassets/mla-corporate/research-and-development/program-areas/livestock-production/20mla-phosphorus-8-page-brochure_apr2021_print.pdf

Mount Sinai (n.d.). *Comfrey.* https://www.mountsinai.org/health-library/herb/comfrey#:~:text=Comfrey%20(Symphytum%20officinale)%20is%20sometimes,inflammation%20and%20keep%20skin%20healthy.

Mount Sinai (n.d.). *Magnesium.* https://www.mountsinai.org/health-library/supplement/magnesium

National Kidney Foundation (n.d.). *Herbal Supplements and Kidney Disease.* https://www.kidney.org/atoz/content/herbalsupp

NC Cooperative Extention (n.d.). *Blackleg in cattle is usually fatal! On ounce of prevention…vaccinate.* https://wilkes.ces.ncsu.edu/2016/07/blackleg-in-cattle-is-usually-fatal-an-ounce-of-prevention-vaccinate/#:~:text=If%20blackleg%20has%20been%20a,a%20few%20hours%20after%20birth.

Nelson, C. (2014, August 22). *Why cattle need vitamin D.* https://www.agproud.com/articles/22552-why-cattle-need-vitamin-d

N Extension (n.d.). *Alfalfa for beef cows.* https://extension.unr.edu/publication.aspx?PubID=2228#:~:text=By%20feeding%205%20pounds%20of,beef%20animal%20for%20less%20cost.

Nickel, R. (2020, February 24). *Critical vitamins for cattle.* https://www.agriculture.com/livestock/cattle/critical-vitamins-for-cattle

Oakland Veterinary (2019, September 27). *Retrospective: A Brief History of Veterinary Medicine.* https://www.ovrs.com/blog/history-of-veterinary-medicine/#:~:text=In%20the%201760s%2C%20Claude%20Bourgelat,animal%20medicine%20predating%209%2C000%20BC.

Partners in Reproduction (n.d.). *Hypocalcemia.* https://www.partners-in-reproduction.com/diseases-disorders/peri-partum-disorders/hypocalcemia/#:~:text=Anorexia%2C%20confusion%2C%20dry%20muzzle%2C,Inability%20to%20urinate

PennState Extension (n.d.). *Minerals for Beef Cows.* https://extension.psu.edu/minerals-for-beef-cows

PennState Extension (2023, March 14). *Herb and Spice History.* https://extension.psu.edu/herb-and-spice-history#:~:text=Herbal%20History&text=Herbs%20are%20mentioned%20in%20Genesis,Europe%20in%20the%20Middle%20Ages.

PennState Extension (2023, July 11). *Cyanide Poisoning of Livestock from Cherry Tree Leaves.* https://extension.psu.edu/cyanide-poisoning-of-livestock-from-cherry-tree-leaves#:~:text=All%20animals%20can%20be%20affected,a%201%2C200%20pound%20dairy%20cow.

Plant Archives (2019). *Effect of adding chamomile to diet and water spraying in milk production and its composition of Holstein cow under heat stress.* https://plantarchives.org/19-2/3467-3472%20(5141).pdf

Progressive Dairy (2020, February 6). *Alternative medicine options for common ailments in cows.* https://www.agproud.com/articles/37037-alternative-medicine-options-for-common-ailments-in-cows

Pubmed (October 10, 2020). *Relationship between Vitamin b12 and cobalt metabolism in domestic ruminant: An update.* https://www.ncbi.nlm.nih.gov/pmc/articles/PMC7601760/#:~:text=Plants%20and%20plant%20products%20contain,natural%20source%20of%20vitamin%20B12.

Rasby, R. (n.d.). *Bloat prevention and treatment in cattle.* https://extensionpublications.unl.edu/assets/html/g2018/build/g2018.htm#:~:text=Bloat%20is%20a%20form%20of,in%20gas%20accumulation%20or%20bloat.

Research Gate (2010, April). *The effect of adding stinging nettle (Urtica dioica) haylage to a total mixed ration on performance and rumen function of lactating dairy cows.* https://www.researchgate.net/publication/259403721_The_effect_of_adding_stinging_nettle_Urtica_dioica_haylage_to_a_total_mixed_ration_on_performance_and_rumen_function_of_lactating_dairy_cows

Riccio, P. (2023, January 4) *Everything You Need To Know About Buttercups.* https://www.southernliving.com/buttercup-flowers-6835625

Salatin, J. (n.d.). *'A Path Toward a Life Worth Living', The Homesteading Guide.* pp. 173-177.

Smaxtec (2020, May 19). *Measuring inner body temperature of dairy cows: An effective method of measuring animal health.* https://smaxtec.com/en/blog/measuring-inner-body-temperature-of-dairy-cows/

Spaulding, C.E. (2010). *Veterinary Guide for Animal Owners.* pp. 14-15

Spaulding, C.E. (2010). *Veterinary Guide for Animal Owners.* pp. 16-43

Spaulding, C.E. (2010). *Veterinary Guide for Animal Owners.* pp. 44-85

Stewart, A. (2022, October). *Hypomagnesemic Tetany in Cattle and Sheep.* https://www.merckvetmanual.com/metabolic-disorders/disorders-of-magnesium-metabolism/hypomagnesemic-tetany-in-cattle-and-sheep#:~:text=In%20the%20most%20acute%20form,of%20the%20eyelids%2C%20and%20nystagmus.

St. Lukes Hospital (n.d.). *Complementary and Alternative Medicine.* https://www.stlukes-stl.com/health-content/medicine/33/000085.htm

Te Pari (n.d.). *Sign, symptoms, and treatment of worms in cattle.* https://www.tepari.com/nz/advice/signs-symptoms-and-treatment-of-worms-in-cattle/#:~:text=The%20most%20common%20types%20of,the%20skin%20by%20larval%20parasites.

The Cattle Site (2022, September 29). *Tetanus in Cattle.* https://www.thecattlesite.com/diseaseinfo/239/tetanus-in-cattle#:~:text=Prevention,as%20possible%20and%20minimise%20contamination.

The Morton Arboretum (n.d.). *Black Cherry.* https://mortonarb.org/plant-and-protect/trees-and-plants/black-cherry/

The Yale Ledger (2022, March 28). *What are the Benefits of Herbal Medicine?* https://campuspress.yale.edu/ledger/what-are-the-benefits-of-herbal-medicine/#:~:text=In%20contrast%2C%20herbal%20medicines%20are,avoid%20their%20possible%20side%20effects.

Understanding Animal Research (n.d.). *Cattle.* https://www.understandinganimalresearch.org.uk/what-is-animal-research/a-z-animals/cattle

University of Kentucky (n.d.). *Using Nutrition to Improve Immunity against Disease in Dairy Cattle: Copper, Zinc, Selenium, and Vitamin E.* https://afs.ca.uky.edu/files/using_nutrition_to_improve_immunity.pdf

University of Massachusetts Amherst (n.d.). *Feeding to reduce phosphorus excretion in dairy cows.* https://ag.umass.edu/crops-dairy-livestock-equine/fact-sheets/feeding-to-reduce-phosphorus-excretion-in-dairy-cows#:~:text=Dairy%20cows%20(and%20the%20rest,more%20phosphorus%20than%20they%20need.

USDA (n.d.). *Poisonous Plant Research.* https://www.ars.usda.gov/pacific-west-area/logan-ut/poisonous-plant-research/docs/milkweed-asclepias-spp/

USDA (n.d.). *Selenium Accumulating Plants.* https://www.ars.usda.gov/pacific-west-area/logan-ut/poisonous-plant-research/docs/selenium-accumulating-plants/

USDA (n.d.). *Water Hemlock.* https://www.ars.usda.gov/pacific-west-area/logan-ut/poisonous-plant-research/docs/water-hemlock-cicuta-douglasii/

USP (2023). *U Publication Herbs SP.* https://www.usp.org/search?search_api_fulltext=publication%20herbs

Zelman, K. (2023, May 2). *What To Know About Nightshade Vegetables.* https://www.webmd.com/diet/what-to-know-about-nightshade-vegetables

www.ingramcontent.com/pod-product-compliance
Lightning Source LLC
Chambersburg PA
CBHW071052290526
45795CB00004B/1448